I0446372

Nursing care

In

Hematology

The Complete Guide

ALEXANDRE CAREWELL

Table of Contents

« Hematology reminds us that in the complex flow of our blood lies the key to life, mystery and healing. »

Chapter 1:
INTRODUCTION TO HEMATOLOGY

The essentials of hematology : definitions and scope

Hematology, a term that at first glance might seem to be reserved for experts, is in fact a medical speciality that we all come into contact with at some point in our lives, if only when we have our blood drawn. Let's take a closer look at this fascinating branch of medicine.

Hematology is the study of blood, the organs that produce it and the diseases that affect it. But it is not limited to these simple definitions. It encompasses a dynamic and complex set of components that interact constantly: the red blood cells that carry oxygen, the white blood cells that defend our body against infection, the platelets that play a key role in coagulation, and plasma, the precious liquid that carries them all.

While blood flows through our veins, guaranteeing our survival and well-being, haematologists strive to decipher the mysteries of this vital fluid. Their research and interventions cover areas as varied as anaemia, coagulation disorders, leukaemia and other blood cancers. The scope of hematology is not confined to a single aspect of medicine. It is at a crossroads, interacting with biology, oncology, genetics and even immunology.

But while hematology is distinguished by its scientific and highly specialised medical nature, it is also profoundly human. Behind every blood sample, every diagnosis, lies a story, an individual, a family. And that's where this speciality comes into its own. Because understanding blood is also understanding life, in all its manifestations, its hopes and its challenges. And it is with this holistic vision that hematology professionals commit themselves every day, for the well-being of their patients, and for the science that is constantly evolving.

Hematology is much more than just the study of blood. It is an ongoing exploration of what makes us living beings, a quest for knowledge that, in turn, leads to better care, better understanding and better living.

History and development of the estate

Hematology, like most medical disciplines, is the product of a long evolution, made up of discoveries, innovations and, above all, insatiable curiosity. Its history is the history of both science and humanity, a journey through the ages where each stage has shaped our current understanding of blood and its mysteries.

Let's go back in time to Antiquity. Long before the terms "red blood cells" or "platelets" entered our lexicon, various civilisations had already identified the central role of blood. For the Egyptians, it was the source of life. For the Greeks, haematos (blood in Greek) was one of the four humours essential to the body's equilibrium. Hippocrates, for example, used this theory of humours to diagnose and treat various illnesses.

But it was during the Middle Ages and the Renaissance that hematology made significant advances. With the emergence of techniques such as dissection, scientists began to dissect human anatomy and gain a better understanding of the circulatory system. It was William Harvey, in the 17th century, who demonstrated that the heart was a pump that propelled blood throughout the body via a closed circuit.

The 19th century marked a major turning point with the invention of the microscope. For the first time, researchers were able to observe blood cells directly, paving the way for crucial discoveries about their form, function and pathology. It was also during this period that doctors such as Rudolf Virchow laid the foundations of modern cellular medicine.

The 20th century was a revolutionary period for hematology. Advances in genetics, molecular biology and technology made it possible to decipher the intimate mechanisms of blood cells, understand diseases such as leukaemia and develop innovative treatments such as chemotherapy.

Today, hematology continues to progress at breakneck speed. From targeted therapies to bone marrow transplants and gene treatments, this field continues to evolve, offering hope and a cure to many patients.

The history of hematology is therefore that of a quest, a passion for knowledge that, century after century, has shaped our understanding of blood and its vital role. And while the road we have travelled is impressive, the future promises many more discoveries, reflecting human ingenuity and determination.

The importance of hematology in the modern medical landscape

Despite its specialisation in blood and blood-related diseases, hematology occupies a central position in the modern medical landscape. Its relevance and importance transcend many borders, making it an essential pillar of the medical world.

At the heart of internal medicine, hematology is at the crossroads of a number of fields. It is inextricably linked with cancerology, with diseases such as leukaemia, lymphoma and myeloma being treated in close collaboration with oncologists. But it also interacts with surgery, particularly when it comes to bone marrow transplants, and with genetics, when the mutations at the root of certain blood disorders are explored.

Hematology is also a key player in emergency medicine. Trauma, surgery or a sudden haemorrhage? Hematology teams are called in to manage blood transfusions, ensure coagulation balance or treat complications such as thrombosis.

It also plays a fundamental role in diagnosis. Who hasn't had a blood test? These analyses, which could be described as routine, are nonetheless essential for assessing a patient's general condition, detecting a disease or monitoring the effectiveness of a treatment. From a simple blood count to more sophisticated tests, diagnostic hematology is often the starting point in the management of many pathologies.

Modern hematology is also at the forefront of innovation. With the emergence of targeted therapies and personalised medicine, it is often at the forefront of introducing and testing new treatments. The study of stem cells, for example, is opening up revolutionary therapeutic prospects, not only for blood diseases, but also for a variety of other pathologies.

But beyond these technical and clinical interactions, hematology also has a profound social impact. Blood donation, the ordinary generosity that saves lives every day, is orchestrated and managed by the field of hematology. In addition, faced with pathologies that are often serious and treatments sometimes lengthy, hematology reminds us of the importance of human accompaniment, listening and support in the care process.

So, far from being just a specialised niche, hematology is in fact a major player, an indispensable link in the vast medical ecosystem. Its role in the modern medical landscape is eloquent testimony to the complexity and interdependence of contemporary medicine.

Chapter 2:
ROLES AND RESPONSIBILITIES
THE HEMATOLOGY NURSE

A versatile profession:
clinical and research role

Within the medical landscape, the role of the haematologist is distinguished by its duality: both front-line clinician and researcher at the cutting edge of innovation. This versatility makes them essential players in the continuum of care, from the patient's bed to the research laboratory.
The Clinical Role

As a clinician, the haematologist is often the first port of call for patients with blood disorders. Whether it's an unexplained anaemia, a sudden thrombosis or a frightening diagnosis such as leukaemia, it's the haematologist's responsibility to make a precise diagnosis, draw up a suitable treatment plan and monitor the patient throughout the course of treatment.

The clinical haematologist works closely with a multidisciplinary team: specialist nurses, laboratory technicians, radiologists, surgeons and many others. Together, they provide holistic patient care, addressing not only the medical aspects, but also the psychological and social needs.

Hematology is a constantly evolving discipline. Blood diseases, in all their diversity and complexity, pose unending enigmas that hematology researchers strive to decipher. These professionals devote themselves to fundamental research, studying the intimate mechanisms of blood cells, or to clinical research, testing new treatments and therapeutic approaches directly on patients.

Research into hematology has led to spectacular advances in recent decades. From targeted therapies to immunotherapies and stem cell transplants, many of these innovations are the result of long hours spent in the laboratory, international collaborations and the unwavering commitment of hematology researchers.
Synergy between Clinical and Research

One of the beauties of the hematology profession lies in this dynamic interaction between the clinic and research. Problems encountered at the patient's bedside often inspire research questions, while discoveries in the laboratory quickly find their way to the wards, improving patients' lives.

Ultimately, this versatility of the haematologist, this ability to oscillate between the world of the patient and that of research, is a testament to the richness and depth of the profession. It also illustrates the commitment of these professionals to pushing back the boundaries of what we know, while ensuring the best possible care for every individual they encounter.

Communication with patients and families

Communication is at the heart of medical practice. In hematology, where diagnoses and treatments can be particularly difficult and complex, the art of communication takes on even greater importance. Talking to a patient or their family requires not only conveying clear information, but also doing so with empathy, respect and compassion.

The Importance of Active Listening
Even before speaking, it is essential to listen. Active listening involves being totally present at the time, without distractions or prejudices. It enables the haematologist to understand not only the patient's symptoms, but also their fears, hopes and concerns. It creates a space of trust where the patient feels valued and heard.

Transmitting clear information
Hematology diseases can be difficult to understand. Complex terms, multiple treatments, variable prognoses... The haematologist must try to simplify this information without diluting it, by presenting it in a structured and accessible way. The use of diagrams, brochures or metaphors can help to make concepts more tangible for patients and their families.

Navigating emotions
A diagnosis in hematology can trigger an avalanche of emotions: shock, denial, anger, sadness... It is essential that the haematologist recognises and validates these emotions. Sometimes, a simple phrase such as "I understand how upsetting this can be" can make a big difference. Emotional support must be offered while guiding the patient through the medical steps ahead.

Encouraging patient participation
Care in hematology is often a collaborative process. Encouraging patients to ask questions, express their preferences or seek clarification strengthens their sense of agency and their involvement in their own health.

Supporting Families
The disease affects not only the patient, but also those around him. Families play a crucial role in support and care. It is therefore essential to include them in conversations, answer their questions and direct them to the appropriate resources if necessary.

Tackling Bad News
Any difficult conversation should be approached delicately. The haematologist should be direct but empathetic,

offering space for emotional reactions while suggesting solutions or next steps.

Ongoing Communication

Communication doesn't stop at the consultation door. Ensuring follow-up, being available for further questions or referring patients to other healthcare professionals for additional support are all elements that strengthen the therapeutic relationship.

Communicating in hematology, as in all areas of medicine, is a delicate balance between transmitting technical information and making a human connection. It's an art that requires listening, patience and, above all, deep humanity.

Interprofessional collaboration: teamwork with doctors, technicians and others

The complex and multi-faceted field of hematology requires close collaboration between different healthcare professionals. This interdependence guarantees optimum patient care, with each specialist contributing his or her expertise to a comprehensive, global vision of care.

<u>Specialist Doctors</u>

Hematology does not work in isolation. It is often at the crossroads of other specialities. These include

- **Oncologists**: For leukaemia, lymphoma and other blood cancers.
- **Rheumatologists**: In the case of autoimmune diseases affecting the blood.
- **Geneticists**: To study the genetic mutations associated with certain blood diseases.

- **Respirologists**: When blood disorders influence or are influenced by lung problems.

This medical collaboration guarantees comprehensive care, with each specialist contributing a piece of the jigsaw.

Laboratory technicians
Technicians are the guardians of blood analysis. They play an essential role in providing accurate and reliable data, which the haematologist then interprets. Their expertise is crucial, because a simple detail in a blood test can guide the diagnosis and treatment plan.

Specialist Nurses in Hematology
They are often on the front line of patient care. Administering treatments, monitoring side effects, or simply offering emotional support, nurses are the daily link between the patient and the medical team.

Pharmacists
With the development of treatments in hematology, drug therapy has become increasingly complex. Pharmacists ensure that medicines are administered correctly, advise on possible interactions, and may even collaborate in the development of targeted therapies.

Social workers and psychologists
The psychological and social dimension of care is essential. Whether it's helping patients deal with the emotional impact of their diagnosis, directing them towards financial resources or simply providing a place to listen, these professionals are essential.

Physiotherapists
Particularly relevant for patients who have undergone surgery, such as transplants, or those requiring rehabilitation following a long period of hospitalisation.

Coordination: the key to success
With so many specialists involved, coordination becomes vital. Regular multidisciplinary meetings, at which each

professional shares his or her observations and concerns, ensure smooth, harmonious care.

Ultimately, if the haematologist can be seen as the conductor of this medical symphony, every musician - be they doctors, technicians, nurses or others - is essential to creating an optimal melody of care for the patient. It is this inter-professional collaboration that ensures that, no matter how complex the case, the patient is always at the centre of attention.

Chapter 3:
MAJOR PATHOLOGIES
IN HEMATOLOGY

Leukaemias: acute and chronic

Leukaemias are a group of blood cancers characterised by an abnormal proliferation of blood cells, mainly white blood cells. They fall into two broad categories: acute and chronic leukaemias, each with its own characteristics and clinical implications.

Acute leukaemia
This type of leukaemia develops rapidly and requires immediate intervention.
- Acute lymphoblastic leukaemia (ALL) :
  - Affects lymphoblasts, immature cells which normally become lymphocytes.
  - It is most common in children, although it can also occur in adults.
  - Symptoms: fatigue, fever, bone pain, bruising and easy bleeding.
- Acute myeloid leukaemia (AML) :
  - Affects myeloblasts destined to become white blood cells (excluding lymphocytes), red blood cells or platelets.
  - It is more common in adults than in children.
  - Symptoms: similar to ALL but may also include joint pain and weight loss.

Chronic leukaemia
These leukaemias progress more slowly and may require no treatment for long periods.
- Chronic lymphocytic leukaemia (CLL) :
  - Affects mature lymphocytes.

- It is the most common form of adult leukaemia in Western countries.
- Symptoms may be absent for a long time. When they do appear, they include fatigue, enlarged lymph nodes and frequent infections.
- Chronic myeloid leukaemia (CML) :
    - Affects the myeloid stem cells of the blood.
    - It is associated with a chromosomal abnormality known as the Philadelphia chromosome.
    - Symptoms include fatigue, weight loss, enlargement of the spleen (splenomegaly) and bone pain.

Care and Treatment
- **Chemotherapy**: Use of drugs to destroy leukaemia cells.
- **Targeted therapy**: use of drugs that target specific abnormalities in leukaemia cells.
- **Bone marrow transplant**: replacement of diseased bone marrow with healthy marrow.
- **Immunotherapy:** Using the immune system to fight cancer.

Leukaemias, whether acute or chronic, represent a challenge in terms of both diagnosis and treatment. With medical advances, the outlook for leukaemia patients continues to improve. It is crucial for hematology carers to understand these diseases in depth, recognise the symptoms and keep up to date with the latest treatments to provide the best possible care for their patients.

Lymphomas :
Hodgkin's and non-Hodgkin's disease

Lymphomas are cancers of the lymphatic system, an essential part of the immune system. They develop when lymphocytes (a type of white blood cell) begin to divide uncontrollably. Lymphomas are generally classified into two broad categories: Hodgkin's lymphoma and non-Hodgkin's lymphoma.

Hodgkin's lymphoma (HL)
- Features:
    - It is defined by the presence of characteristic cells called Reed-Sternberg cells.
    - It generally has a predictable pattern of spread from one group of lymph nodes to another.
- Symptoms:
    - Painless enlargement of lymph nodes, unexplained fever, night sweats, weight loss, itching.
- Subtypes:
    - Classical HL (which includes several sub-categories such as lymphocytic nodularity, nodular sclerosis, etc.).
    - Lymphocytic LH.

- Treatments:
    - Chemotherapy, radiotherapy, targeted therapy and immunotherapy.

Non-Hodgkin's lymphoma (NHL)
- Features:
    - NHL is a heterogeneous group of lymphomas which do not contain Reed-Sternberg cells.
    - They can be either B-cell or T-cell.

- Symptoms:
  - Although similar to HL, the symptoms of NHL are often less specific. They include enlarged lymph nodes, abdominal pain and fatigue.
- Subtypes:
  - There are more than 60 different subtypes of NHL. Some of the most common include diffuse large B-cell lymphoma, follicular lymphoma and marginal zone lymphoma.
- Treatments:
  - Treatment depends on the type and stage of the lymphoma. It may include chemotherapy, radiotherapy, targeted therapy, immunotherapy and sometimes stem cell transplantation.

Differentiation Factors

- **Age and sex**: Although both types of lymphoma can occur at any age, HL is more common in young adults and people over the age of 55. NHL is more common in older adults.
- **Location and spread**: HL often spreads in an orderly fashion from one group of lymph nodes to another, whereas NHL can appear anywhere and spread unpredictably.
- **Growth rate**: Some NHLs may grow slowly and not require immediate treatment, while others may be aggressive and require rapid intervention.

Lymphomas, although grouped under the same name, present a wide variety in terms of presentation, course and treatment. Understanding the nuances between Hodgkin's lymphoma and non-Hodgkin's lymphomas is crucial to the accurate diagnosis and appropriate management of patients. With advances in modern medicine, many lymphoma patients can now look forward to a complete remission or a prolonged life with the disease.

Coagulation disorders and platelet diseases

Coagulation disorders and platelet diseases are conditions that affect the blood's ability to clot normally, leading to an increased risk of bleeding or, conversely, excessive clotting. These disorders can result from a variety of causes, ranging from genetic mutations to acquired diseases.

Coagulation disorders
These disorders are often due to a deficiency or malfunction of one or more coagulation factors.
- Haemophilia:
    - **Haemophilia A**: caused by factor VIII deficiency.
    - **Haemophilia B**: results from a factor IX deficiency.
    - Symptoms: prolonged bleeding after injury, internal haemorrhage, haematomas, joint pain due to internal bleeding.
- Von Willebrand disease:
    - An inherited condition in which the blood lacks a clotting protein called von Willebrand factor or it does not function properly.
    - Symptoms: nasal bleeding, bleeding gums, heavy periods, easy bruising.
- Thrombophilia:
    - Refers to an abnormal propensity to thrombosis. There are several forms, including antiphospholipid syndrome and factor V Leiden mutation.
    - Can lead to blood clots in the veins and arteries.

Platelet Diseases

Platelets are small fragments of blood cells which play an essential role in coagulation.

- Thrombocytopenia:
    - A low platelet count which may be due to reduced platelet production, increased platelet destruction or a combination of both.
    - Common causes: aplastic anaemia, cirrhosis, myelodysplastic syndrome, certain viral infections.
- Thrombotic thrombocytopenic purpura (TTP):
    - A rare condition in which small blood clots form in the blood vessels.
    - Symptoms: purpura (small bruises under the skin), fatigue, fever, confusion.
- Thrombocytosis:
    - An abnormally high platelet count, which may be reactive (in response to an underlying condition) or due to a bone marrow disorder, such as polycythaemia vera.
- Platelet dysfunction:
    - When platelets do not function properly, often due to hereditary diseases or certain medications.

Management and processing

- Coagulation disorders can often be managed with replacement treatments that replace the missing coagulation factor.
- Platelet diseases may require platelet transfusions, immunosuppressive drugs, or treatments to address the underlying cause.
- Management will depend largely on the specific diagnosis, the severity of the condition and the patient's individual needs.

Coagulation disorders and platelet diseases present a complex set of clinical challenges. A thorough understanding of these conditions is crucial to their proper management. With the development of treatments and a better understanding of these diseases, many patients are now able to lead normal, active lives.

Anemia : from origin to care

Anemias are a group of diseases in which the blood's ability to carry sufficient oxygen to the tissues is impaired, generally due to a low haemoglobin level or an insufficient number of red blood cells. They can have several causes, and their management largely depends on the underlying cause.

Classification and Origins of Anemia
- Anemia due to deficiency:
    - **Iron deficiency anaemia**: caused by a lack of iron, often due to blood loss (such as heavy periods) or reduced iron absorption.
    - **Megaloblastic anaemia**: resulting from a vitamin B12 or folate deficiency.
- Haemolytic anaemia:
    - Red blood cells are destroyed faster than the bone marrow can produce them.
    - Causes: infections, autoimmune diseases, genetic disorders such as hereditary spherocytosis.
- Aplastic anaemia:
    - The bone marrow does not produce enough red blood cells.
    - May be triggered by medication, infection or be idiopathic (with no known cause).
- Haemoglobinopathic anaemia:
    - Caused by genetic mutations affecting the structure or production of haemoglobin.

- Examples: sickle cell anaemia, thalassaemia.

Common symptoms
- Fatigue
- Pallor
- Shortness of breath
- Palpitations
- Headaches
- Dizziness or lightheadedness

Diagnosis

Diagnosis of anaemia usually begins with a blood test called a complete blood count (CBC). Depending on the results, further tests may be required, such as serum ferritin, vitamin B12, folate, or other specialist examinations to determine the cause.

Management of anaemia
- Anemia due to deficiency:
    - **Iron deficiency anaemia:** iron supplements and treatment of the underlying cause (e.g. stopping bleeding).
    - **Megaloblastic anaemia**: vitamin B12 injections or oral folate supplements.
- Haemolytic anaemia:
    - Treatment of the underlying cause, for example drugs for an infection or immunosuppressants for an autoimmune disease.
- Aplastic anaemia:
    - Immunosuppressants, blood transfusions or bone marrow transplants in severe cases.
- Haemoglobinopathic anaemia:
    - Sickle cell disease: analgesics, hydration, blood transfusions, hydroxyurea.
    - Thalassaemia: regular blood transfusions, iron chelation to prevent overload.

31

Anemias are a heterogeneous group of diseases, each requiring a specific approach to diagnosis and management. Early detection and appropriate management can help improve patients' quality of life and prevent potentially serious complications. With an in-depth knowledge of the different types of anaemia, healthcare professionals can offer their patients optimal care.

Chapter 4:
TECHNIQUES
AND SPECIFIC PROCEDURES

Blood transfusions :
types, complications,
and special considerations

Blood transfusions are common medical procedures involving the administration of blood components from a donor to a recipient. These transfusions can save lives in a variety of situations, including after surgery, trauma or for patients suffering from certain blood diseases.

Types of blood transfusion
- **Red blood cell transfusion**: Used to treat anaemia, blood loss following surgery or trauma, and certain blood diseases.
- **Platelet transfusion**: For patients with low platelet counts, such as those with leukaemia, cancer or who have received chemotherapy.
- **Plasma transfusion**: Plasma is the clear liquid in blood, containing electrolytes, water and proteins. It can be transfused in cases of coagulation disorders.
- **Granulocyte transfusion**: Rarely used, but may be necessary for some patients with severe infection and low granulocyte counts.
- **Cryoprecipitates and coagulation factors**: Used to treat certain coagulation disorders.

Complications of blood transfusions
- **Allergic reactions:** Mild symptoms such as itching or skin rashes, but can sometimes be serious.

- **Haemolytic reactions**: When the body attacks transfused blood, which can be dangerous or even fatal.
- **Fluid overload**: Can occur if blood is transfused too rapidly, especially in patients with compromised cardiac function.
- **Transmission of infections**: The risk is very low thanks to rigorous testing, but infections such as hepatitis and HIV can theoretically be transmitted.
- **Reaction to platelet transfusion**: Non-haemolytic febrile reactions are common with platelet transfusions.

Special Considerations
- **Blood types**: Compatibility between different blood types (A, B, AB, O) and Rh factors (+ or -) is essential to avoid haemolytic reactions.
- **Auto-transfusion**: Where a patient donates their own blood prior to planned surgery, to be transfused afterwards if necessary.
- **Irradiated blood**: Prevents a rare complication called "graft-versus-host disease". It is often used for immunocompromised patients.
- **Transfusions for Jehovah's Witnesses**: Some people refuse blood transfusions for religious reasons, requiring alternative approaches.
- **Storage of blood**: Blood and its components have a limited shelf life.
- **Specific blood products**: Some patients, such as those with rare antibodies, may require specially selected blood.

Blood transfusions are a cornerstone of modern medicine, saving countless lives. Although generally safe, they come with a unique set of risks and considerations. A thorough understanding of these aspects is essential for healthcare professionals to ensure that transfusions are as safe and effective as possible.

Bone marrow biopsies : preparation and post-operative care

A bone marrow biopsy is a medical procedure that extracts and examines a small sample of bone marrow, usually from the hip bone. It is essential for diagnosing and monitoring many blood diseases and other conditions.

Preparation for a Bone Marrow Biopsy
- Preliminary consultation:
  - Discussion with the doctor about the reasons for the biopsy, the potential benefits and the associated risks.
  - Review of the patient's current medication, as some, such as anticoagulants, may need to be modified or discontinued.
- Fasting:
  - The patient may be asked to fast for several hours before the procedure to minimise the risk of aspiration, especially if sedation is planned.

- Consent:
  - Signing a consent form after fully understanding the risks and benefits.
- Clothing and jewellery:
  - Wear comfortable clothing and avoid jewellery or other metal objects.

The procedure
- Positioning:
  - The patient generally lies on his or her side or stomach.
- Local anaesthetic:

- The puncture site, often the posterior iliac bone, is anaesthetised using an injection.
- Puncture:
  - A special needle is inserted into the bone to take a sample of liquid marrow (aspiration) and/or a small bone fragment containing marrow (biopsy).

Post-operative care
- Surveillance:
  - After the procedure, the patient is observed for a short period to detect any signs of complications or side effects.
- Pain management:
  - It is normal to feel some pain or discomfort after the procedure. Over-the-counter or prescribed painkillers may be used.
- Wound care:
  - The puncture site must be kept clean and dry for 24 hours. A sterile dressing may be applied and should be changed as directed.
- Activity:
  - It is generally advisable to rest for the rest of the day. Normal activities can generally be resumed the following day.
- Signs of complications:
  - Although rare, complications can include infection, prolonged bleeding or a build-up of blood in the puncture site. It is essential to consult a doctor if signs of infection (redness, heat, swelling, purulent discharge) appear, or if the pain worsens.

Bone marrow biopsy is a valuable diagnostic procedure that requires appropriate preparation and post-operative care to ensure patient safety and comfort. Communication between the healthcare professional and the patient is essential to minimise anxiety, clarify expectations and ensure optimal recovery.

Cellular therapies and stem cell transplants

Cell therapies and stem cell transplants are innovative medical interventions that exploit the potential of cells to treat, and sometimes cure, a multitude of diseases. In hematology, they are mainly used to treat malignant and non-malignant blood disorders.

Cellular therapies
- **Definition**: Cellular therapies encompass the use of cells to treat or prevent a disease. These cells may come from the patient (autologous) or from a donor (allogeneic).
- **CAR-T cells**: A recent innovation in which a patient's own T cells are modified in the laboratory to attack cancer cells, then reinjected into the patient. Mainly used for certain types of leukaemia and lymphoma.
- **Dendritic cells**: These cells can be used to stimulate an immune response against cancer by presenting tumour antigens to T cells.

Stem cell transplants
- **Definition**: This involves replacing stem cells that are diseased or destroyed by chemotherapy or radiotherapy with healthy stem cells.
- Stem cell sources:
    - **Bone marrow:** Traditionally the main source of stem cells.
    - **Peripheral blood: An increasingly** common source after special stimulation to increase the number of stem cells in the blood.
    - **Umbilical cord blood:** Rich in stem cells and used, albeit less commonly, for transplants.

- Types of grafts:
  - **Autologous**: The stem cells come from the patient themselves, harvested before intensive treatment and then reinjected.
  - **Allogeneic**: The stem cells come from a donor. This may be a family member, an identical twin or an unrelated donor.
- **Conditioning**: Before the transplant, the patient undergoes intensive chemotherapy, with or without radiotherapy, to destroy the diseased bone marrow. This is a crucial stage, but can lead to a number of complications.
- **Graft rejection**: A major concern, especially with allogeneic transplants. The recipient's immune system may attack the transplanted stem cells, or conversely, the transplanted cells may attack the recipient's tissues (graft-versus-host disease).

Benefits and challenges
- **Curative potential**: These therapies can offer a chance of cure for otherwise incurable diseases.
- **Limitations and risks**: Potential side effects and risks associated with conditioning chemotherapy, post-transplant complications, and logistical and financial challenges.

Cell therapies and stem cell transplants represent hope for many patients suffering from blood diseases. Their complexity requires in-depth understanding and specialist training, but constant advances in the field continue to expand their possibilities and perfect their techniques.

Chapter 5:
COMPLICATION MANAGEMENT

Sign recognition and symptoms of complications

Early recognition of the signs and symptoms of complications is essential to intervene quickly and ensure the best chance of recovery for hematology patients. After procedures such as chemotherapy, radiotherapy or stem cell transplantation, the immune system is often weakened, leaving the patient vulnerable to a range of complications.

1. Infections:
   - **Symptoms**: Fever, chills, sweating, coughing, shortness of breath, pain or burning when urinating, redness, heat or swelling of a wound.
   - **Action**: Fever may be the only sign of infection in immunocompromised patients. Any sign of infection should be treated as an emergency.
2. Graft-versus-host disease (GVHD):
   - **Symptoms**: Skin rash or desquamation, diarrhoea, jaundice or icterus, muscle or joint pain, dry eyes or mouth.
   - **Action**: Start immunosuppressive treatment or adapt current treatment.
3. Thrombosis:
   - **Symptoms**: Pain, swelling, redness or warmth in a leg or arm. Difficulty breathing, chest pain, palpitations or fainting may indicate a pulmonary embolism.
   - **Action**: Anticoagulants and close monitoring are required.
4. Toxicity of chemotherapy and radiotherapy:
   - **Symptoms**: Nausea, vomiting, hair loss, fatigue, mouth ulcers, diarrhoea or constipation.

- **Action**: Adjust doses, administer supportive medication or change treatment regime.
5. Anemia:
   - **Symptoms**: Fatigue, paleness, shortness of breath, dizziness, palpitations.
   - **Action**: Blood transfusion, erythropoietin or other bone marrow stimulating drugs may be considered.
6. Haemorrhage or bleeding:
   - **Symptoms**: easy bruising, bleeding gums, blood in Feces or urine, prolonged bleeding from small cuts.
   - **Action**: Platelet transfusions, vitamin K or other treatments to promote coagulation.
7. Reaction to transfusion:
   - **Symptoms**: Chills, fever, hives, chest pain, shortness of breath.
   - **Action**: Stop the transfusion immediately and inform the medical team.

Early recognition and management of complications in hematology are crucial to patient prognosis. Patient and family education is also essential. They need to know what symptoms to look out for and understand the importance of alerting the healthcare team quickly. Close collaboration between the patient, their family and healthcare professionals is the key to navigating this complex area and ensuring the best outcomes.

Infection management in immunocompromised patients

Managing infections in immunocompromised patients is a fundamental aspect of hematology care. These patients, because of their underlying condition or the treatments they are receiving (such as chemotherapy), have weakened immune systems, making them particularly vulnerable to infection.

1. Assessment and monitoring :
   - **Medical history**: Determine risk factors, recent treatments, exposures and travel.
   - **Clinical examination**: Look for signs of infection, particularly in common sites such as the lungs, urine, skin and blood.
   - **Laboratory tests**: blood cultures, urine cultures, liver function tests, complete blood count, and other specific tests depending on the symptoms.
2. Prophylaxis :
   - **Prophylactic antibiotics**: In some patients, prophylaxis may be recommended to prevent bacterial, fungal or viral infections.
   - **Vaccinations**: Although some live vaccines are contraindicated in immunocompromised patients, others, such as inactivated influenza vaccine, may be beneficial.
3. Processing :
   - **Empirical therapy**: Start antibiotics quickly in febrile patients without waiting for culture results.
   - **Targeted therapy**: Adjust treatment according to the results of cultures and sensitivity tests.
   - **Patient isolation**: Limiting the spread of infection to other vulnerable patients.
4. Management of complications :
   - **Sepsis**: A systemic inflammatory response to infection that can lead to septic shock and organ failure. Rapid intervention is essential.
   - **Antibiotic resistance**: Monitor closely and adapt treatment if necessary.
5. Education and prevention :
   - **Hand hygiene**: Regular and thorough hand hygiene is the most effective preventive measure.
   - **Avoiding exposure**: Patients should avoid sick people, crowds or areas where they are more likely to be exposed to pathogens.

- **Diet**: Encourage a diet that minimises the risk of exposure to pathogens, such as avoiding raw or undercooked foods.
6. Psychosocial support :
- **Anxiety and depression**: Fear of infection can be a source of anxiety. Psychological support and interventions can help manage these concerns.

Infections in immunocompromised patients can be severe and potentially life-threatening. Close monitoring, rapid intervention and comprehensive education of patients and carers are crucial to prevent and manage these infections. The medical team, in collaboration with the patient, must be constantly vigilant and proactive in the fight against infections.

Pain and relief in hematology

Pain is a complex and subjective experience, influenced by biological, psychological and social factors. In hematology, pain can result from the disease itself, from the treatments administered or from associated complications. Appropriate pain management is essential to improve patients' quality of life and their ability to tolerate treatment.

1. Understanding pain in hematology :
- **Causes of pain**: Tumour expansion, obstruction, inflammation, infection or the side-effects of treatment can all be sources of pain.
- **Types of pain**: acute vs. chronic, nociceptive vs. neuropathic, somatic vs. visceral.
2. Pain assessment :
- **Assessment scales**: Use of standardised tools such as the visual analogue scale (VAS) or the numerical scale.

- **History of pain**: duration, location, radiation, characteristics, aggravating or alleviating factors, and associated symptoms.

3. Pharmacological strategies :
   - **Non-opioid analgesics**: Paracetamol, non-steroidal anti-inflammatory drugs (NSAIDs).
   - **Opioids**: Morphine, fentanyl, oxycodone, etc. Adjustments for tolerance, dependence and side effects.
   - **Adjuvants**: Antidepressants, anticonvulsants, corticosteroids for neuropathic pain or other specific types of pain.

4. Non-pharmacological interventions :
   - **Physical therapies**: physiotherapy, massage, application of heat or cold.
   - **Complementary therapies**: Acupuncture, biofeedback, meditation and relaxation.
   - **Psychological support**: counselling, support groups, cognitive-behavioural therapy to manage the stress and anxiety associated with pain.

5. Special considerations in hematology :
   - **Bone pain**: Common in diseases such as multiple myeloma. May require palliative radiotherapy or bisphosphonates.
   - **Neuropathic pain:** often the result of chemotherapy or tumour invasion of the nerves.
   - **Pain associated with procedures**: bone marrow biopsies, lumbar punctures, insertion of central catheters.

6. The challenges of pain management :
   - **Fear of dependence**: Educate patients about the distinction between dependence and tolerance.
   - **Side-effects**: Constipation, nausea, confusion, often requiring simultaneous management.
   - **Cultural or social barriers**: Respecting and understanding beliefs and attitudes towards pain and its treatment.

Pain in hematology is a challenge that requires a holistic and personalised approach. Recognising pain, correctly assessing its nature and intensity, and implementing an appropriate care plan are essential. Collaboration between the patient, family and healthcare team is crucial to ensuring effective relief and improving quality of life.

Chapter 6:
EMOTIONAL CHALLENGES
AND PSYCHOLOGICAL

Coping with serious diagnoses: support tools and techniques

Dealing with a serious diagnosis, such as a haematological malignancy, is an unsettling and potentially traumatic time for the patient and their family. As a hematology nurse, it is crucial to have the tools and techniques to support these patients through this difficult medical journey.

1. Active listening and empathy :
   - **Listening without judgement**: Set aside time to listen to the patient's concerns and feelings.
   - **Empathy**: Recognising and validating the patient's emotions, showing understanding and support.
2. Provide clear information :
   - **Simple explanations**: use accessible language and avoid medical jargon.
   - **Information on demand**: some patients want to know all the details, others prefer an overview. We adapt to their needs.
3. Relaxation and stress reduction techniques :
   - **Deep breathing**: A simple but effective technique for reducing anxiety.
   - **Meditation and mindfulness**: Helping patients to focus on the present moment and distance themselves from their worries.
4. Psychosocial support :
   - **Referral to specialists**: Psychologists, social workers or psychiatrists for further support.

- **Support groups**: These groups provide a space where patients can share their experiences with others in similar situations.

5. Advanced planning and discussions on end of life :
   - **Advance directives** : Helping patients to define their wishes regarding future care.
   - **Honest discussions**: Talking about difficult subjects such as prognosis, palliative care and the end of life.

6. Involving family and friends :
   - **Education and resources**: Providing families with information about the disease, treatments and how they can support the patient.
   - **Support groups for families**: Providing a space where loved ones can also share their concerns and learn from others.

7. Self-management strategies :
   - **Journaling**: Encourage patients to write about their experiences, which can provide an outlet and perspective.
   - **Creative activities**: Painting, music or dance can offer ways of expressing emotions and managing stress.

8. Use of technology :
   - **Well-being and meditation applications**: A number of applications can help patients practise meditation or other relaxation techniques.
   - **Forums and social networks**: Some patients find comfort in talking to other people in similar situations around the world.

Dealing with a serious diagnosis requires a multi-dimensional approach that goes far beyond medical treatment. As a nurse, understanding and being equipped to support the emotional, psychological and social dimensions of the illness is essential to improving the patient's quality of life and supporting them as best they can through this ordeal.

Support at the end of life and mourning

Support at the end of life and bereavement are fundamentally human stages, marked by intense vulnerability. These moments give rise to profound reflections on life, death and the impact of our existence. For a hematology nurse, these moments are poignant encounters with the reality of the human condition.

When a patient with terminal hematology disease is admitted, the therapeutic approach changes. It is no longer a question of fighting the disease, but of celebrating life while respecting imminent death. In this context, the relationship between carer and patient is transformed. The touch, the look, the silence and the spoken word take on a new depth. Medical gestures become gestures of love, respect and homage to the dignity of the person.

Patients and their families are often trying to make sense of the end of life. The nurse's comforting presence and sympathetic ear can help them explore these existential questions. They provide a safe space in which to express fears, regrets, hopes and goodbyes. This role of facilitator is essential, as it enables each person to find inner peace and accept the inevitable.

But support does not stop at the moment of death. The death of a patient echoes in the hearts of those left behind. The family, plunged into mourning, must face up to the absence and rebuild a life without their loved one. Here again, the nurse has a role to play. By their discreet presence, they can support loved ones in the grieving process, direct them to appropriate resources or simply offer a shoulder to cry on.

Death, however painful, is an integral part of our existence. It reminds us of our fragility, but also of the inestimable value of every moment we live. Support at the end of life and bereavement are not only experiences of loss, but also of love, resilience and rebirth. And for nurses, they are a reminder of the nobility of their mission: to be at the service of life, at every stage.

Stress management and prevention burnout for professionals

Managing stress and preventing burnout are major issues for healthcare professionals. The constant pressure, immense responsibilities and heavy emotions associated with serious diagnoses or the loss of patients can lead to physical, emotional and mental exhaustion. In a hematology department, where diseases are often complex and the stakes of life and death are palpable, these challenges take on an even more significant dimension.

Nurses and healthcare professionals are often compared to marathon runners. But even the toughest runner needs breaks, recovery and support to avoid overload and exhaustion. The first step is to recognise that stress is not a simple weakness, nor is it inevitable. It is the product of a combination of individual, professional and organisational factors.

Awareness is essential. Recognising the early signs of burnout, such as chronic fatigue, irritability, reduced empathy or a drop in performance, means you can take action before it's too late. It's also vital to understand that taking care of yourself is not a luxury, but a necessity. Relaxation, hobbies, regular breaks from work and a healthy lifestyle are all ways of recharging your batteries.

Communication is another key element. Talking about your emotions, concerns or doubts with colleagues, superiors or outside professionals can ease the burden of everyday life. Mutual support between colleagues is also invaluable, as it creates an environment where everyone feels understood and supported.

On an organisational level, stress management training, discussion groups and relaxation areas can be set up. Recognition for a job well done, caring management and appropriate working hours can also contribute to greater well-being at work.

Finally, it's essential to keep in mind why you chose this profession in the first place. Reconnecting with your original vocation, the desire to help and care, can help you get through the difficult times.

Stress management and burnout prevention for healthcare professionals are essential to ensure not only their well-being, but also optimal patient care. In an environment as demanding as hematology, this requires constant attention, mutual support and a commitment to continuous improvement.

Chapter 7:
ADVANCES AND INNOVATIONS IN HEMATOLOGY

Clinical research : ongoing trials and implications for the nurse

Clinical research spearheads medical advances. In hematology, a field rich in therapeutic innovations, clinical trials play an essential role in the discovery of new treatments and approaches to combat various blood diseases. But where do nurses fit into this dynamic?

Nurses are, in fact, at the heart of the implementation of clinical trials. They are the bridge between the patient and the research team. Their role is varied, ranging from data collection to patient education and the administration of experimental treatments.

The nurse's first responsibility is patient safety. Above all, they must ensure that the patient fully understands the nature of the trial, the potential benefits and risks, and that they give informed consent. Understanding the trial protocol, drug doses, frequency of administration and potential side effects is essential.

The nurse also plays a crucial role in data collection. Rigour is essential. Any change, whether in the patient's condition, in the side effects experienced or in other relevant observations, must be precisely recorded. This data is vital for assessing the efficacy and safety of the treatment being tested.

Communication is also central. The nurse is often the first point of contact for the patient. They must be able to explain the nature of the trial, answer questions, allay concerns and offer emotional support. They also act as an intermediary between the patient and the research team, ensuring that any concerns or complications are quickly addressed.

Ongoing training is also a requirement for nurses involved in clinical research. Trial protocols are evolving, new treatments are emerging, and nurses need to keep their knowledge up to date to ensure the best possible patient care.

Finally, ethics are fundamental. The rights, safety and well-being of patients are paramount. Nurses must ensure that the integrity of the trial is maintained, while putting the patient at the centre of their concerns.

In conclusion, nurses play a major role in carrying out clinical trials in hematology. They ensure that the trial runs smoothly, guarantee patient safety and contribute to the progress of medicine. Their role is both complex and rewarding, as they play an active part in the advent of new therapeutic approaches that will improve patients' lives.

Gene and targeted therapies : personalised medicine

21st century medicine is undergoing an unprecedented transformation thanks to the emergence of gene and targeted therapies. The generalist approach to medical treatment, in which the same treatment was prescribed to all patients suffering from the same pathology, is gradually giving way to personalised medicine. This medical revolution is particularly marked in hematology, where the potential of these new approaches is enormous.

Gene therapy aims to introduce, remove or genetically modify material within an individual's cells to treat a disease. For example, in the case of a genetic disease where a gene is defective, gene therapy can make it possible to introduce a healthy copy of this gene to restore the cell's normal function. In the context of hematology, gene therapies are being studied for diseases such as haemophilia and certain forms of anaemia.

Targeted therapies, on the other hand, have been designed to specifically target diseased cells while sparing healthy cells. These therapies exploit molecular differences between diseased cells (such as cancer cells) and normal cells. For example, some targeted therapies in hematology target proteins specifically expressed by leukaemia cells, thereby stopping their growth or eliminating them directly.

Personalised medicine stems from these innovations. It recognises that each patient is unique and that their disease, even if it has the same name as another patient's, may have very different characteristics at the molecular level. The treatment of two leukaemia patients, for example, may vary according to the genetics and molecular characteristics of their cancer cells.

These advances offer great hope, but they also bring new challenges. The cost of these therapies is often high, and their availability can be limited. What's more, their implementation requires in-depth training for healthcare professionals and close collaboration between clinicians, researchers and laboratories.

For hematology nurses, this means keeping abreast of the latest advances, understanding the mechanisms of action of these therapies, and being able to explain these complex treatments to patients and their families. They must also be alert to the specific side-effects of these new therapies and be able to manage them.

Gene and targeted therapies are redefining the landscape of medicine and offering innovative therapeutic prospects for many hematology diseases. Nurses, who are at the heart of these developments, have a fundamental role to play in guaranteeing the efficacy and safety of these treatments, while ensuring that patients receive individualised, humane care.

The future of hematology : from expectations to hopes

Hematology, a medical discipline devoted to the study of blood, bone marrow and the diseases that affect them, is at the crossroads of major innovations. From genomic sequencing to immunotherapy, hematology is preparing for promising advances that could radically transform the way we diagnose, treat and think about blood diseases. With this future in mind, it is essential to understand both what we expect from the future and the hopes that are driving the field.

Technological and clinical expectations
- **High-throughput genomic sequencing:** With the advent of ever more powerful sequencing techniques, we expect to gain a better understanding of the genetic abnormalities at the root of many hematology diseases. This detailed knowledge will make it possible to identify new therapeutic targets and develop tailor-made treatments.
- **Regenerative medicine:** Advances in stem cell biology could pave the way for the regeneration of damaged tissues or organs, offering new options for conditions such as severe anaemia or medullar aplasia.

- **Innovations in transplants:** We hope to improve bone marrow transplant techniques, reduce complications and extend this therapeutic option to a greater number of patients thanks to more widely available compatible donors.

Hope for patients and society
- **Less invasive treatments:** The hope is to develop therapies that are both more effective and less distressing for the patient, minimising side effects while maximising efficacy.
- **A better quality of life:** As well as treating the diseases themselves, the aim is to offer patients a better quality of life, by managing symptoms, reducing pain and providing adequate psychological support.
- **Accessibility and equity:** The hope is that every patient, regardless of location or financial situation, can benefit from the best treatment options available. This requires global collaboration to ensure equitable access to treatment.
- **Education and awareness:** As the field evolves, it is essential to raise public awareness of advances in hematology, encourage blood and bone marrow donation, and invest in the education of healthcare professionals.

The future of hematology is bright, driven by technological advances and a collective desire to improve patients' lives. There are still many challenges ahead, but with close collaboration between researchers, clinicians, patients and decision-makers, hematology is well on the way to achieving its greatest aspirations.

Chapter 8:
PRACTICAL ADVICE AND RESOURCES FOR HEMATOLOGY NURSES

Further training : training and seminars

The medical world, with its constant advances in research, technology and clinical care, requires professionals to constantly update their skills. For hematology nurses, further training is more than a necessity: it's a vocation. Dedication to clinical excellence, to the patient and to the art of care requires continuous learning. In this chapter, we explore the importance of training and seminars for the hematology nurse.

Why is continuing training essential?
- **Evolving knowledge**: The field of hematology is constantly evolving. New discoveries are made, innovative therapies are introduced and protocols are updated.
- **Improving clinical skills**: In-depth training enables nurses to acquire new skills, develop existing ones and keep abreast of best practice.
- **Patient safety**: By keeping abreast of the latest methods and recommendations, nurses can guarantee optimal, safe patient care.
- **Professional fulfilment**: Continuing training fosters confidence, expertise and career advancement.

Types of training and seminars
- **Clinical training**: Focused on practical skills, this covers subjects such as the administration of chemotherapy, palliative care and biopsy techniques.
- **Research seminars**: These sessions provide updates on advances in hematology research, including new treatments, clinical trials and scientific discoveries.

- **Communication workshops**: These courses focus on non-technical but essential skills, such as communicating with patients, teamwork and stress management.
- **Webinars and online training**: Thanks to technology, many educational resources can now be accessed remotely, offering flexibility and diversity in the subjects covered.
- **Congresses and conferences**: These large-scale events offer the opportunity to network with other professionals, exchange knowledge and learn from world experts.

Optimising the training experience
- **Planning**: Identify your training needs, set yourself objectives and look for the opportunities that best match your aspirations.
- **Active engagement**: Take an active part in the sessions, ask questions and engage in discussions.
- **Practical application**: Apply what you learn as soon as possible to consolidate your knowledge.
- **Knowledge sharing**: pass on what you've learned to your colleagues, creating a collective learning environment.

The road to excellence in hematology is an ongoing journey. Through regular training and a commitment to learning, hematology nurses can not only enhance their clinical practice, but also enrich their careers and, above all, provide the best possible care for their patients.

Tools and applications to make it easier daily practice

In a world dominated by technology, digital tools and applications have become invaluable companions for healthcare professionals, including hematology nurses. These tools can simplify many aspects of daily practice, from patient management to continuing education and inter-professional communications. Here's a look at the innovations that are transforming hematology nursing practice.

Patient Management and Medical Follow-up
- **Electronic Medical   Records (EMR)**: These provide rapid, secure access to patient information, ensuring optimum coordination of care.
- **Treatment monitoring applications**: These tools help patients keep track of their medication, side effects and appointments, while giving nurses a real-time overview.
- **Teleconsultation   platforms**: These allow patients to be consulted remotely, which is particularly useful for monitoring patients who are immunocompromised or geographically remote.

Communication and collaboration
- **Secure messaging systems**: Communicate confidentially with colleagues, share clinical information or discuss cases.
- **Videoconferencing   platforms**: For team meetings, remote training or discussions with specialists.

Training and Educational Resources
- **Continuing education applications**: These offer learning modules, videos, quizzes and other resources to keep you up to date.
- **Digital libraries**: Access to research articles, professional journals and up-to-date clinical guidelines.
- **Specialist   podcasts and webinars**: For on-the-go training, covering a variety of hematology topics.

Time Management and Organisation
- **Digital   diaries**: schedule appointments, tasks and reminders.

- **Notes and** to-do **lists applications**: For jotting down important information, ideas or tasks.
- **Stress management and well-being tools:** guided meditation, breathing techniques and mood monitoring to support carers' mental health.

Other Practical Tools
- **Medical converters and calculators**: for drug dosages, unit conversions or indices specific to hematology.
- **Drug interaction applications**: to quickly check the compatibility of treatments.
- **Patient information tools**: To provide patients with clear and reliable information about their conditions, treatments and care.

By integrating these tools and applications into their daily practice, hematology nurses can improve the efficiency, safety and quality of the care they provide. However, it is crucial to always ensure data confidentiality and compliance with standards of care. With the right training and judicious use, these technological innovations can truly transform modern nursing practice.

Support networks and professional associations

Support networks and professional associations play a crucial role in the field of hematology and for the nurses who work in it. Not only do they provide professional and emotional support, they are also a valuable source of education, knowledge sharing and networking opportunities. Let's find out how these structures enhance the work of the hematology nurse.

The importance of Support Networks
- **Knowledge exchange**: Forums, discussion groups and meetings enable nurses to share their experiences, tackle complex cases and learn from each other.
- **Emotional Support**: Healthcare professionals, particularly in demanding specialties such as hematology, can be faced with stressful situations. Having a network to discuss, vent or seek advice from is invaluable.
- **Mentoring and coaching**: Newcomers to the industry can benefit from the advice and guidance of experienced professionals.

Professional Associations: A Pillar for Nurses
- **Continuing Education and Training**: These associations often organise workshops, conferences and webinars on current and relevant topics.
- **Lobbying and Representation**: They can defend nurses' rights, influence health policy or propose improvements in professional practice.
- **Resources and Publications**: Access to specialist journals, clinical guidelines and other professional resources.
- **Networking opportunities**: The conferences and events organised by these associations offer a unique opportunity to meet colleagues, establish professional contacts and learn more about advances in the field.

Some Renowned Associations
- **The International Society of Hematology**: dedicated to promoting and disseminating knowledge about blood diseases.
- **Association of Nurses in Hematology and Oncology**: specifically for nurses, it offers training, resources and a support network.

- **Local support groups**: In many countries or regions, there are specific associations or support groups dedicated to hematology.

For hematology nurses, it is essential to actively engage with support networks and professional associations. Not only do they provide valuable resources for clinical practice, but they also offer a community of peers with whom to share, learn and grow. Ultimately, by relying on these networks, nurses can improve their care delivery, personal wellbeing and professional careers.

Chapter 9:
PATIENTS AND THEIR FAMILIES :
COMPREHENSIVE CARE

The importance of the relationship carer in hematology

The care-giver-patient relationship is an essential pillar in all areas of medicine. In hematology, where patients are often faced with serious diagnoses and long and sometimes complex treatments, this relationship takes on a particularly profound and significant dimension. Let's find out why this relationship is so crucial in hematology.

The Vulnerability of Hematology Patients
Hematology patients are often faced with life-threatening diseases such as leukaemia, lymphoma or other blood disorders. Their medical course may involve invasive procedures such as bone marrow biopsies, recurrent blood transfusions or even stem cell transplants.

- **Need for information**: These patients need clear communication about their diagnosis, treatment options and their implications. Understanding their illness and its treatment helps them to cope better with this difficult period.
- **Intense emotions**: Fear, anxiety, anger and sometimes even guilt can emerge. An understanding and supportive Caregiver can help navigate through these feelings.

The nurse: a constant point of reference
Nurses are often the main point of contact for patients, being present at every stage of the medical process.

- **Mutual trust**: Patients need to trust their nurse to feel safe and follow treatment recommendations.

Conversely, the nurse must trust the patient to follow instructions and express concerns.
- **Active listening**: Hematology nurses need to be trained in active listening, providing a space where patients can express their fears, hopes and concerns.

Humanity and Empathy
Empathy is essential in the carer-patient relationship. Every patient is unique, and understanding their personal, cultural and social situation is crucial.
- **Beyond the disease**: seeing the patient not just as a disease to be treated, but as a person with aspirations, dreams and fears.
- **Support** : In the darkest moments, such as when a relapse or complications are announced, the empathetic presence of a carer can offer invaluable support.

Impact on Medical Outcomes
A good caregiver-patient relationship can even influence medical outcomes.
- **Adherence   to treatment**: A patient who feels supported and understood is more likely to follow the treatment plan.
- **Early detection of complications**: Open communication enables early detection of side effects or complications.

The caregiver-patient relationship in hematology is a delicate dance between medical science and humanity. It is a partnership based on mutual trust, empathy and respect. In a field where the stakes are so high, the quality of this relationship can make all the difference, both to the patient's well-being and to the effectiveness of the treatment. For hematology nurses, investing time and effort in this relationship is not only a professional obligation, but also a unique opportunity to make a difference to the lives of their patients.

Educating patients and their families about the disease and its treatment

Educating patients and their families about the disease and treatment is a central role of the hematology nurse. This education is crucial not only for a better understanding of the disease, but also to ensure compliance with treatment, manage expectations and reduce anxiety. Here is an overview of this essential aspect of care.

Diagnosis: A turning point for the patient and the family
The news of a diagnosis of hematology, whether leukaemia, lymphoma or another blood disorder, can turn the world of the patient and their family upside down. Emotions flood in - shock, denial, fear, confusion.

- **The first stage**: The nurse must provide clear information about the illness itself, its cause, its possible course and its implications.
- **Language**: It is crucial to use language that is adapted to the patient's and family's level of understanding, avoiding overly complex medical jargon.

Understanding Treatment
Treatment in hematology can be long, complex and sometimes painful.

- **Treatment options**: Each disease may have several therapeutic approaches. The nurse explains the different options, their advantages, disadvantages and potential side effects.
- **Duration and plan**: Patients need to have an idea of the timetable - how long the treatment will last, how many hospital visits will be required, etc.

Managing side effects
Most hematology treatments have side effects.

- **Preventive information**: Before starting treatment, inform the patient of the common side-effects and how to manage them.
- **Warning signs**: Underline any symptoms or reactions that require immediate medical attention.

Family involvement
Actively involving the family in the educational process has many advantages.
- **Emotional support**: An informed family can offer more appropriate support to the patient.
- **Practical help**: The family can help manage medication, recognise side effects or provide transport to hospital.

Teaching Resources and Materials
The use of brochures, videos or reliable websites can supplement verbal explanations.
- **Visual aids**: Diagrams, models or animations can help explain complex concepts.
- **Support Groups**: Directing patients and families to local support groups or patient associations can provide a platform for exchange and sharing.

Educating patients and their families is a holistic approach. It is not just about passing on medical information, but also about reassurance, establishing a relationship of trust and actively involving the patient in their own care. It's a huge responsibility, but also an opportunity for nurses to have a profound impact on the lives of patients and their families, by guiding them through the challenges of illness and treatment.

The cultural and ethical dimension in hematology

The cultural and ethical dimensions of hematology transcend mere medical practice. These aspects, which are sometimes neglected or underestimated, can have a profound influence on the way patients are cared for and their experience of the disease. So how do these dimensions manifest themselves in hematology, and how can healthcare professionals be sensitive to them?

The Cultural Dimension in Hematology
- **Diversity of beliefs**: Patients come from a range of cultures, religions and traditions. Each culture has its own perception of illness, health, life and death.
- **Traditional practices**: Some patients may use traditional remedies or cultural rituals alongside their medical treatment. Understanding and respecting these choices is crucial.
- **Communication**: Language barriers can be a problem. Having access to interpreters or translated resources is essential to ensure clear and effective communication.
- **Dietary considerations**: Certain cultural or religious diets may have implications for patient nutrition, particularly during treatment.

Ethical Issues in Hematology
- **Informed Consent**: Ensure that patients fully understand the implications of their treatment, the associated risks and the other options available.
- **Confidentiality**: Respect for privacy and the confidentiality of patients' medical information are paramount.
- **End of life and palliative care**: Decisions concerning the end of life, in particular the cessation of treatment or the introduction of support measures,

must be taken with sensitivity, taking into account the wishes of the patient and his or her family.
- **Access to care**: In certain contexts, access to expensive or cutting-edge treatments can raise ethical questions, particularly about the way in which these resources are allocated.

Integrating Culture and Ethics into Clinical Practice
- **Continuing education**: Nurses and other healthcare professionals should receive continuing education on cultural and ethical issues.
- **Active listening**: Take the time to listen to patients' concerns, beliefs and values.
- **Ethics committees**: Having access to hospital ethics committees can help navigate complex or ambiguous situations.
- **Inclusion policies**: Promoting a culture of inclusion and diversity within medical institutions ensures that patients' cultural needs are recognised and respected.

Like all medical fields, hematology is not limited to biology or physiology. It lies at the intersection of science, culture and ethics. By recognising and respecting the cultural and ethical dimension of care, healthcare professionals can offer more holistic, empathetic and personalised care, responding not only to patients' physiological needs, but also to their emotional, spiritual and cultural needs.

Chapter 10:
SPECIFIC PHARMACOLOGY
IN HEMATOLOGY

Essential medicines : indications, contraindications and side effects

Medicines used in hematology cover a wide range of pathologies, from simple anaemia to more complex blood cancers such as leukaemia or lymphoma. It is essential that nurses understand the indications, contraindications and side effects of the medicines they administer. Here is a summary of some of the key drugs in hematology, although this is only a fraction of those available.

1. Alkylating agents (e.g. Cyclophosphamide)
   - *Indications*: Treatment of several cancers, including leukaemia, lymphoma and myeloma.
   - *Contraindications*: Known allergies, certain kidney or liver disorders.
   - *Side-effects*: Bone marrow suppression, nausea, hair loss, kidney toxicity.
2. Antimetabolites (e.g. methotrexate)
   - *Indications* : Acute leukaemia, lymphoma.
   - *Contraindications*: Pregnancy, breast-feeding, severe hepatic or renal insufficiency.
   - *Side-effects*: Liver toxicity, mouth ulcers, diarrhoea.
3. Anti-tumour antibiotics (e.g. Doxorubicin)
   - *Indications* : Various cancers, including certain lymphomas.
   - *Contraindications*: Heart failure, rhythm disorders.
   - *Side-effects*: Cardiac toxicity, hair loss, myelosuppression.

4. Supporting agents (e.g. Epoetin)
  - *Indications* : Anemia associated with chronic renal failure or chemotherapy.
  - *Contraindications*: Uncontrolled hypertension, history of thrombosis.
  - *Side-effects*: Hypertension, risk of blood clots, joint pain.
5. Tyrosine kinase inhibitors (e.g. Imatinib)
  - *Indications* : Chronic myeloid leukaemia, certain other cancers.
  - *Contraindications*: Known allergy to the drug.
  - *Side-effects*: oedema, nausea, skin rashes, muscle pain.
6. Corticosteroids (e.g. Prednisone)
  - *Indications*: Several hematology pathologies, such as Hodgkin's disease, chronic lymphocytic leukaemia.
  - *Contraindications*: Active untreated infections, peptic ulcers.
  - *Side-effects*: Increased appetite, insomnia, mood swings, long-term osteoporosis.

This overview of essential medicines in hematology highlights the need for healthcare professionals to have a thorough understanding of pharmacology. Hematology drugs can be potent with significant side effects. Cautious administration, careful monitoring and adequate patient education are essential to ensure patient safety while maximising treatment efficacy.

Advances in targeted therapies

Targeted therapies have revolutionised the treatment of hematology diseases. Unlike traditional chemotherapy, which attacks all rapidly dividing cells indiscriminately, targeted therapies specifically attack the molecules involved in the growth and survival of cancer cells. This reduces the damage caused to healthy cells, offering a more tolerable side-effect profile.

1. Tyrosine Kinase Inhibitors (TKIs)
   - *Example*: Imatinib, used mainly for chronic myeloid leukaemia (CML).
   - *Mechanism of action*: These drugs block the activity of protein tyrosine kinases, which play an essential role in cell signalling and cancer cell growth.
   - *Advantages*: A long-lasting response with a relatively mild side-effect profile, particularly when compared with traditional chemotherapy.
2. BCL-2 inhibitors
   - *Example*: Venetoclax, used for chronic lymphocytic leukaemia (CLL).
   - *Mechanism of action*: BCL-2 is a protein that prevents cancer cells from dying. Venetoclax inhibits this protein, causing cancer cells to die.
   - *Benefits*: Remarkably effective, especially when combined with other therapies.
3. Inhibitors of the PI3K/AKT/mTOR pathway
   - *Example*: Idelalisib, used for certain types of lymphoma.
   - *Mechanism of action*: Targets the PI3K pathway, essential for the survival and proliferation of cancer cells.
   - *Benefits*: Provides a new option for patients resistant to other treatments.
4. PARP inhibitors
   - *Example*: Olaparib, used in certain solid cancers, but also being explored for leukaemia.
   - *Mechanism of action*: Prevents cancer cells from repairing their DNA, leading to their death.
   - *Advantages*: Particularly effective in patients with certain genetic mutations.
5. Immunoconjugation therapies
   - *Example*: Brentuximab vedotin, for the treatment of Hodgkin's lymphoma.

- *Mechanism of action*: combines a specific antibody with a toxin. The antibody targets a protein on cancer cells, delivering the toxin directly to the cell.
- *Benefits*: Precise attack on cancer cells, minimising damage to healthy cells.

Advances in targeted therapies offer new hope to patients suffering from hematology diseases. They enable more specific treatments, reduce side effects and can be used either alone or in combination with other therapies. Research in this field is dynamic, with the hope of discovering new targets and developing even more effective therapies.

Administration and management of medicines : precautions and best practices

The administration and management of medicines is a crucial part of the nursing role, particularly in hematology where patients can receive complex and powerful treatments. Medication errors can have serious consequences, so it's essential to follow rigorous practices to ensure patient safety.

1. The "Five Good Ones
This is a fundamental rule of drug administration:
- *Good patient* : Always check the patient's identity.
- *The right medicine* : Make sure you have the right medication.
- *Correct dose*: Check that the dose is correct.
- *Correct route*: Confirm that you are using the correct route of administration (oral, IV, etc.).
- *The right time*: Administer the medicine at the right time.

2. Understanding the medicine
   - Know the drug, its indications, contraindications, potential side effects and drug interactions.
   - Be aware of medicines that require special dilution or administration over a period of time.
3. Adequate preparation
   - Prepare medicines in a calm, uninterrupted environment to minimise errors.
   - Use precise measuring devices for liquid medicines.
4. Patient monitoring
   - Monitor the patient for allergic reactions or side effects after administration.
   - Know the patient's basic vital signs before administration, particularly if the drug may influence these parameters.
5. Full documentation
   - Document immediately after administration.
   - Include the name of the drug, dose, route, time and any relevant observations.
6. Effective communication
   - Inform the patient about the medicine they are about to receive, its purpose and potential side effects.
   - Contact the care team if you have any concerns or anomalies.
7. Precautions with high-risk drugs
   - Medicines such as chemotherapy require specific precautions, such as the use of personal protective equipment during preparation and administration.
   - Some medicines may require close monitoring of the patient, such as regular blood sampling.
8. Continuing Education
   - Keep up to date with new recommendations, changes in protocols or the introduction of new drugs.
9. Encouraging patient participation
   - Well-informed patients can be active partners in their own care. Encourage them to ask questions and report any adverse effects.

10. Be close to the pharmacy
   • Establish good communication with the pharmacy department, as pharmacists are an invaluable resource for questions relating to medicines.

The safe administration of medicines is essential to ensure the well-being of patients. This requires a combination of knowledge, attention to detail, good practice and communication. In the field of hematology, with its complex, targeted therapies, these precautions are even more crucial.

Chapter 11:
PATIENT QUALITY OF LIFE

The challenges of everyday life and adapting to illness

Living with a hematology disease can present multidimensional challenges, from physical symptoms to emotional upheaval. For patients and their families, adapting to the disease often means reshaping daily life and reassessing priorities.

1. Physical symptoms and limitations
   * **Fatigue**: One of the most common symptoms, fatigue can severely limit daily activity. It's not just a feeling of drowsiness, but a profound exhaustion that doesn't always improve with rest.
   * **Pain**: Chronic pain can be a reality, requiring both drug and non-drug management.
   * **Side-effects of treatment**: Nausea, hair loss and neuropathy, among others, can affect quality of life.
2. Emotional and psychological adaptations
   * **Fear and anxiety**: Fear of the progression of the disease, of treatments or of the unknown is common. Therapy sessions, support groups and relaxation techniques can help.
   * **Depression**: Faced with illness, some people may feel a sense of powerlessness or persistent sadness.
   * **Self-esteem**: Body changes and limitations can influence self-perception.
3. Social and relational impact
   * **Isolation: Because of** their symptoms or the need to protect their immune system, some patients may feel isolated.

- **Family dynamics**: Roles within the family may change. A spouse or child may become a carer, for example.
- **Intimate relationships**: Illness and treatment can affect libido and body image, influencing intimate relationships.

4. Professional challenges
- **Work capacity**: Depending on the severity of the disease and the effects of treatment, it may be necessary to reduce working hours or take medical leave.
- **Discrimination at work**: Although illegal in many countries, some patients may experience discrimination because of their illness.

5. Practical adaptations
- **Diet and nutrition**: A healthy diet can help manage certain symptoms and boost immunity.
- **Exercise**: Appropriate exercise can improve strength, endurance and mental well-being.
- **Planning**: Having a calendar for medical appointments, medication and rest can help structure the day.

6. Financial aspects
- **Medical costs**: Treatments, consultations and medication can be expensive, even with insurance.
- **Loss of income**: If the patient or carer has to work less or stop working, this can have an impact on household income.

Adapting to life with a hematology disease is a journey, not a destination. Every patient and family will navigate these challenges differently. Help is available in many forms, from medical professionals to support groups and complementary therapies. The key is to seek support, ask questions and remember that you don't have to face these challenges alone.

Rehabilitation and physiotherapy for hematology patients

Rehabilitation and physiotherapy play a crucial role in the management of patients with hematology-related diseases. Although these diseases primarily target the blood and lymphatic system, their impact on the body can be vast and multidimensional, requiring integrative therapeutic approaches to improve the patient's quality of life.

1. Rehabilitation: An Overview
Rehabilitation aims to help patients regain or maintain an optimal level of physical, emotional and social functioning, despite the challenges imposed by the disease.
- **Initial assessment**: This involves a full assessment of the patient's level of function, including mobility, strength, endurance, pain, respiratory capacity and emotional well-being.
- **Individualised objectives**: Based on the assessment, specific, achievable objectives are set for each patient.

2. Physiotherapy
- **Improving mobility**: Patients may suffer from joint stiffness or muscle weakness due to inactivity, especially after long periods in hospital. Physiotherapists help with joint mobilisation and muscle strengthening.
- **Pain management**: Techniques such as thermotherapy, cryotherapy, ultrasound or manual therapy can be used to manage pain.
- **Respiratory therapy**: Some patients may require breathing exercises to improve lung capacity, especially if they have had lung infections or if the disease affects lung function.

3. Activities of Daily Living (ADL)

Occupational therapists work with patients to help them resume activities of daily living, such as dressing, cooking, or even more complex tasks such as returning to work.

4. Emotional and Social Adaptation

Rehabilitation is not just about the body. Social workers, psychologists and other professionals can help patients adapt emotionally to their illness, manage anxiety and depression, and navigate social challenges such as returning to work or adjusting to family life.

5. Patient education

It is crucial that patients understand their illness, their treatments and how these can affect their bodies. Education can help them to take an active part in their rehabilitation.

6. Group Workshops

These workshops can cover topics such as nutrition, stress management, adapted physical activity, etc. They also provide an opportunity for patients to discuss and support each other.

7. Long-term monitoring

Rehabilitation does not stop when patients leave hospital. Regular monitoring ensures that patients continue to make progress and adapt to their daily lives.

Rehabilitation and physiotherapy are essential to ensure optimal quality of life for patients suffering from hematology diseases. By taking into account the whole person, these interventions aim to restore function, self-confidence and autonomy, enabling patients to live life to the full despite their illness.

Nutrition and dietetics in hematology

Nutrition plays a fundamental role in the management of patients suffering from hematology diseases. A balanced and appropriate diet can not only help to alleviate some of the side effects of treatment, but also strengthen the immune system, improve healing and promote general well-being.

1. Why is Nutrition Crucial?
   - **Treatment support**: Hematology treatments, particularly chemotherapy, can be extremely hard on the body. Appropriate nutrition provides essential energy and nutrients to support the body during this period.
   - **Boosting the immune system**: A balanced diet can help boost the immune system, which is crucial for hematology patients who may be more susceptible to infections.
2. Nutritional challenges in hematology
   - **Loss of appetite**: Common with some treatments, this may be due to nausea, changes in taste or other side effects.
   - **Digestive disorders**: Nausea, vomiting, diarrhoea or constipation may occur.
   - **Increased energy requirements**: Fighting illness can increase the body's energy requirements.
3. Dietary recommendations
   - **Protein**: Crucial for tissue repair and construction, as well as immune function. Sources: lean meat, fish, eggs, legumes, dairy products.
   - **Carbohydrates:** Provide energy. Favour complex carbohydrates such as wholegrain cereals.
   - **Fats**: Opt for healthy sources such as avocados, nuts, olive oil and oily fish.
   - **Vitamins and Minerals**: Crucial for healing and immune function. A varied diet is key.

4. Hydration

Hydration is essential, particularly to help eliminate toxins and medications from the body.

5. Foods to avoid

- **Unpasteurised or raw foods: Because of** the increased risk of infection.
- **Alcohol**: May interact with certain medicines and weaken the immune system.
- **Very sweet or salty foods**: Can exacerbate certain side effects such as water retention.

6. Practical advice

- **Eat smaller meals**: If loss of appetite is a problem, opt for smaller, more frequent meals.
- **Calorie enrichment**: If weight gain is difficult, enrich meals with nutritional supplements.
- **Supplements**: To be discussed with the doctor or dietician. Some may be beneficial, while others may interfere with treatment.

7. Working with a dietician

- **A dietician specialising** in oncology or hematology can provide tailored advice and help draw up a tailor-made nutritional plan.

Nutrition in hematology is a cornerstone of treatment and recovery. Every patient is unique, so it's essential to have the right advice, to listen to your body and to work closely with healthcare professionals to ensure optimal nutrition throughout your treatment.

Chapter 12:
CLINICAL CASES
AND SITUATION STUDIES

Analysis of complex cases
and how to respond

Hematology is a complex field, with patients often presenting with polymorphic symptoms and diagnoses that require a multidimensional approach. In this chapter, we will explore the analysis of complex cases in hematology, focusing on the methodology of approach and resolution of these situations.

1. Understanding Complexity
- **Multiple symptoms**: A patient may present with a combination of symptoms that do not clearly correspond to a single disease.
- **Drug interactions**: Hematology patients are often taking several drugs, which may interact with each other or with the disease itself.

2. Approach Methodology
- **Gathering information**: Take a detailed history, including medical history, medication, current symptoms and their progression.
- **Clinical examination**: It is essential to carry out a thorough physical examination, paying attention to subtle clinical signs.
- **Investigations**: Laboratory tests, biopsies and medical imaging, among others, can provide essential information.

3. Solving Complex Cases

- **Interprofessional collaboration**: Involving specialists from other medical disciplines can bring a different perspective or specialist skills.
- **Literature review**: In some cases, it may be useful to search the medical literature for similar cases or evidence-based recommendations.
- **Colleague consultation**: Discussing the case with colleagues or at clinical meetings may bring new ideas or similar experiences.
- **Regular follow-up**: In some cases, the diagnosis may not be immediately obvious. Close monitoring of the patient allows us to observe the evolution of symptoms and adjust the diagnostic approach.

4. Examples of complex cases

- **Leukaemia with Atypical Neurological Symptoms**: How to differentiate between complications of the disease, side effects of medication or another concomitant pathology?
- Refractory Anemia with Excess Blasts (RAEB) in the Context of Other Autoimmune Disease: How can both conditions be managed simultaneously without exacerbating one or the other?

5. The Importance of Communication

- **With the patient**: Clearly explain the uncertainties, the next steps and reassure the patient while remaining transparent.
- **With the family**: Keep the family informed, especially when they are involved in the patient's care.
- **With the Care Team**: Ensuring clear and regular communication with all members of the care team to ensure coordinated care.

Complex cases in hematology challenge the diagnostic and therapeutic skills of healthcare professionals. However, with a methodical approach, close collaboration between professionals, and transparent communication with patients and their families, these challenges can be met, leading to optimal patient care.

Common ethical dilemmas and reflections

Ethical dilemmas are situations where it is difficult to determine the best action to take because of conflicting moral or ethical principles. In hematology, where decisions can influence quality of life, length of life, or even life itself, these dilemmas are common. Let's look at some of these ethical dilemmas and the thinking that goes into them.

1. Interruption of Treatment at the End of Life
Dilemma: When, or if, should you stop a treatment that prolongs life but could also reduce its quality?
Reflection: Balancing the principle of "do no harm" with that of offering the best possible quality of life. Listening to the wishes of the patient and their family, while drawing on expert advice.

2. Full disclosure to the patient
Dilemma: How far to disclose details of a serious diagnosis or prognosis to a patient?
Reflection: Striking a balance between the patient's right to information and the protection of their emotional and mental well-being.

3. Clinical Research on Patients
Dilemma: How do you recruit patients for clinical trials without unduly influencing their decision or compromising their well-being?

Reflection: Ensuring informed consent, ensuring that patients understand the risks and benefits, and guaranteeing that their participation is entirely voluntary.

4. Distribution of Limited Resources
Dilemma: How do you allocate resources (such as a bone marrow transplant) when demand outstrips supply?
Reflection: Use ethically defensible criteria for distribution, such as the probability of success, while avoiding any form of discrimination.

5. Respect for Patient Autonomy vs. the Best Interest
Dilemma: What do you do when a patient refuses life-saving or life-prolonging treatment?
Reflection: Respect the patient's autonomy while ensuring that they fully understand the consequences of their choice.

6. Decisions on Incapacitated Patients
Dilemma: How do you make decisions for patients who cannot express their wishes, such as those in a coma or suffering from mental health problems?
Reflection: Rely on a legal representative or an advance directive, and always act in the patient's best interests.

7. Confidentiality vs. Risk to Others
Dilemma: What if a hematology patient poses a risk to others (e.g. a contagious disease) but does not want this to be disclosed?
Reflection: Balancing the patient's right to confidentiality with the protection of public health.

Ethical dilemmas in hematology require careful thought, open communication and inter-professional collaboration. It is essential to remember that each patient is unique, and that there is not always a 'right' answer. The aim is to strive to make decisions that respect both ethical principles and the individual needs of the patient.

Feedback :
lessons learned from daily practice

The day-to-day practice of hematology is a complex mix of science, art and humanity. While textbooks can teach theory, it is the patient's bedside that offers the most valuable lessons. Here's a look at what hematology nurses have to say, highlighting the invaluable lessons learned from day-to-day practice.

1. Patience is a Virtue
In hematology, patients often go through long and trying treatments. It is essential to learn to be patient, not only in waiting for results, but also in managing patients' expectations and emotions.

2. Active Listening is Crucial
Patients can sometimes give subtle clues about their condition or their concerns. Learning to really listen - without interrupting or assuming - can lead to a better diagnosis, a better understanding and a better therapeutic relationship.

3. Each Patient is Unique
Two patients with the same diagnosis may have very different symptoms, responses to treatment and emotional needs. Treating each patient as an individual is fundamental.

4. Self-care is Essential
The emotionally charged nature of hematology can lead to burnout. Learning to look after yourself, recognise the

signs of fatigue and seek support is crucial to longevity in the field.

5. Ethics Above All
Faced with ethical dilemmas, many professionals have learned the importance of being well informed about ethical principles, seeking advice and always acting in the patient's best interests.

6. Effective Communication is the Key
Whether with colleagues, patients or their families, clear and effective communication avoids misunderstandings, fosters trust and improves results.

7. Learning Never Stops
Medicine is constantly evolving. Hematology nurses have found that keeping up to date with the latest research, technology and best practice is essential.

8. Compassion is the Heart of the Profession
When faced with a serious diagnosis, compassion is often what helps patients get through the difficult times. The ability to offer compassion without becoming emotionally overwhelmed is a valuable skill.

9. Teamwork is Invaluable
Hematology is a multidisciplinary field. Working effectively with other specialists, whether doctors, technicians or consultants, improves patient care.

10. Celebrating Small Victories
In a field where the challenges are many, appreciating the small victories - whether a symptomatic improvement or good news on examination - brings joy and renewal to daily practice.

Hematology, with its challenges and rewards, offers countless learning opportunities. Lessons learned from daily practice, grounded in real experience, are essential to guide and inform the next generation of professionals.

Chapter 13:
THE LEGAL FRAMEWORK AND ETHICS

Patients' rights in hematology

Patients' rights in hematology, as in any other medical field, are of paramount importance in ensuring fair, respectful and patient-centred care. This care aims not only to treat the disease, but also to respect the patient's dignity, autonomy and preferences. Here is a fluid exploration of these rights:

The Foundations of Patients' Rights
Hematology is a specialised field of medicine that deals with often complex and life-threatening diseases. In this context, the importance of patients' rights is accentuated. These rights form the basis of the relationship of trust between patient and healthcare professional, and are a guarantee of high-quality care.

Right to Information
Every patient has the right to be informed in a clear and comprehensible manner about his or her state of health, the proposed treatments, their benefits and risks, and other possible alternatives. This information enables patients to make informed decisions about their health.

Informed Consent
Before any intervention or treatment, patients must give their consent. They must be informed of the implications, risks and potential benefits. In hematology, where treatments such as chemotherapy or bone marrow transplants can have severe side effects, this consent is crucial.

Data confidentiality
A patient's medical information is confidential. It cannot be shared without the patient's consent, except in exceptional circumstances provided for by law.

The right to privacy and respect
Patients have the right to be treated with dignity and respect, without discrimination. This includes respect for their privacy during examinations and treatment.
Right to a Second Opinion
If a patient has doubts or concerns about their diagnosis or treatment, they have the right to seek a second opinion from another specialist.
Active participation in the Care Plan
Patients have the right to be actively involved in the planning and implementation of their care plan. They can accept or refuse treatment, and have the right to be informed of the implications of these decisions.
The right to quality care
Every patient has the right to receive the best possible medical care, in line with current standards and guidelines.
Access to medical records
Patients have the right to access their medical records and to receive copies if necessary.
Right to lodge a complaint
If a patient feels that their rights have not been respected, they have the right to lodge a complaint.

Recognising and respecting the rights of hematology patients is not just an ethical and legal obligation for healthcare professionals; it is essential to ensuring patient-centred care. These rights aim to balance the power dynamic between professional and patient, placing the patient at the heart of all decisions concerning his or her health.

Responsibilities
and obligations of the nurse

Nurses play a central role in patient care, acting as a link between the patient and the medical team. They perform a variety of essential functions, ranging from direct care to educational, administrative and research duties. Here is a fluid presentation of nurses' responsibilities and duties:

A Central Role in the Care Process

The nurse's position at the crossroads of multiple interactions means that he or she is the guarantor of comprehensive, personalised patient care. But with this central role comes a heavy responsibility.

Direct Patient Care

It's probably the first image that springs to mind: the nurse at the patient's bedside. This responsibility encompasses administering medication, caring for wounds, taking vital signs, as well as assessing the patient's pain and emotional well-being.

Education and advice

Nurses have a duty to inform and educate patients and their families about their illness, its treatment, what to do and how to prevent it. The aim of this education is to empower patients and improve their quality of life.

Care Coordination

Nurses coordinate care between different healthcare professionals, guaranteeing continuity and consistency of care. They can act as a link between the doctor, physiotherapist, psychologist and other specialists.

Needs Assessment

Nurses regularly assess the patient's state of health, detect any complications and adjust care accordingly. This ongoing assessment is essential to anticipate and respond to the patient's changing needs.

Rigorous documentation

Nurses must meticulously document each treatment, intervention or observation in the patient's medical file. This traceability is crucial for patient safety, care coordination and legal liability.

Respect for ethics and patients' rights
Every patient must be treated with dignity, respect and without discrimination. Nurses also ensure that medical information is kept confidential.

Continuing Professional Development
Nurses have a duty to keep up to date with medical advances, care techniques and regulations. This ongoing training obligation guarantees high-quality care based on the latest scientific evidence.

Interprofessional collaboration
Nurses work closely with a multidisciplinary team. This collaboration requires communication, mutual respect and the sharing of skills to ensure optimum patient care.

Resource Management
Nurses manage the material and human resources at their disposal to provide care. This management must be effective in order to guarantee patient safety and well-being, while optimising costs.

The scope and complexity of the nursing profession require dedication, skill and humanity. In addition to techniques and knowledge, it is also a profession guided by a strong ethic, centred on the respect and well-being of the patient. The responsibilities and obligations of nurses are therefore both a burden and an honour, reflecting the crucial importance of this profession in the healthcare system.

Protocols and standards in hematology: ensuring compliance

Hematology is a complex and constantly evolving discipline, requiring care based on precise protocols and standards. These protocols are essential to guarantee safe and effective patient care. They evolve in line with new scientific discoveries and clinical practice.

Protocols and Standards in Hematology: Why are they Necessary?

Hematology, at the crossroads of biology and clinical practice, demands the utmost precision. Every detail counts. Protocols and standards guarantee this accuracy, enabling every patient to benefit from care based on the best available evidence.

Research-based protocols

Hematology is an active field of research. New therapies, new diagnostic methods and new approaches to care are regularly being developed. Hematology protocols are based on these discoveries, adapting to the cutting edge of science.

Patient Safety Assurance

Patient safety is paramount. By following precise protocols, the risks of errors, drug interactions or complications are minimised. It's also a guarantee of quality care.

Standards for uniform practice

Hematology standards ensure a degree of uniformity in patient care, whatever the institution or practitioner. They serve as a common reference, facilitating dialogue and collaboration between professionals.

Ensuring Compliance: A Daily Challenge

The implementation of protocols and standards requires constant vigilance. Several steps are essential to ensure compliance:

- **Continuing education**: All healthcare professionals, whether nurses, doctors or laboratory technicians, need to keep abreast of the latest developments in protocols and standards.
- **Internal audits**: Healthcare institutions carry out regular audits to check that clinical practice complies with current standards.
- **Feedback**: Teams are encouraged to share their feedback to identify potential deviations from protocols and take the necessary corrective action.

- **Regular Protocol Updates**: Protocols are reviewed on a regular basis, ensuring that they reflect the latest scientific advances and feedback from the field.
- **Digital tools**: Institutions are increasingly relying on digital tools to make it easier to monitor protocols, automatically report anomalies or non-conformities, and ensure traceability of care.

Compliance with hematology protocols and standards is not an end in itself, but a means of ensuring the best possible patient care. It is the reflection of evidence-based medicine, attentive to the needs of each individual patient, and constantly striving for improvement.

Chapter 14:
CAREER DEVELOPMENT IN HEMATOLOGY

Specialisation opportunities and advancement

The hematology nursing profession is both demanding and rewarding. As with any medical profession, the learning never really stops, because medical science is constantly evolving. For those who are passionate about this field, there are several routes open to them, allowing them to specialise further or climb the ladder in the medical world.

Starting out as a hematology nurse means entering a complex world where every day brings its own challenges. It's a world that demands an in-depth knowledge of human physiology, innovative treatments, and an ability to establish empathetic relationships with patients. But with this solid foundation, the door opens to even more advanced specialisations.

Some may choose to focus on specific pathologies, such as acute leukaemia or lymphoma, becoming experts in these particular fields. Others may be attracted by the technical side and decide to specialise in performing bone marrow biopsies or administering complex cell therapies.

As these skills develop, leadership opportunities may emerge. Clinical nurse specialists or nurse managers may supervise teams, play a role in training newcomers, or even participate in setting up clinical protocols in their institution.

Research is another exciting avenue. With treatments and therapeutic approaches constantly evolving, taking part in clinical trials or observational studies can be a route to advancement for those who are curious and keen to make a tangible contribution to medical science.

Finally, teaching is an area where experienced nurses can really shine. By passing on their knowledge to the next generation, they play an essential role in training competent and compassionate future professionals.

While hematology already offers a wealth of knowledge and experience, the opportunity to specialise further or move up the professional ladder adds another dimension to this career. Whether it's out of passion for a specific field, professional ambition, or the simple desire to help others, the horizons in hematology are vast and promising.

Hematology research for nurses: getting involved and making a contribution

Research in hematology offers a vast range of opportunities and discoveries. It is the driving force behind medical progress, enabling the emergence of new therapies and improved management protocols. Although doctors and scientists are often on the front line, the role of nurses in this field is just as crucial. The involvement of nurses in hematology research offers them not only the opportunity to develop professionally, but also to make an active contribution to the development of care.
A Key Position in Clinical Research

Nurses are often the first to observe the side effects of treatments, to perceive patients' needs or to identify practical aspects that could be improved. These daily observations, combined with appropriate training and supervision, can lead to relevant research questions. By taking part in clinical trials, nurses can play a key role in collecting data, administering new treatments or monitoring patients.

Getting involved: how to get started
To get involved in research, nurses can start by approaching a university hospital or clinical research unit. Taking part in specific research training courses, attending seminars or joining working groups are all ways of acquiring skills and becoming familiar with the research environment.

Interdisciplinary collaboration
The strength of research lies in collaboration. Working closely with doctors, pharmacologists, biologists and other healthcare professionals means that perspectives can be cross-fertilised and projects enriched. Nurses bring a unique vision, focused on the patient and his or her overall care, which can guide research into areas that are sometimes neglected.

Contributing to scientific literature
As well as actively participating in studies, nurses can also contribute to the scientific literature. Writing articles, sharing feedback or presenting work at conferences are all ways of disseminating knowledge and promoting the role of nurses in research.

Research as a Vehicle for Professional Development
Getting involved in research can also open the door to career opportunities. Becoming a research nurse coordinator, getting involved in larger-scale projects or even pursuing a doctorate are all possible prospects.

Research in hematology is not limited to laboratories or leading researchers. It draws on the curiosity, expertise and passion of everyone, including nurses. By getting involved, nurses can not only enrich their career paths, but also actively contribute to shaping the future of hematology care.

Mentoring and training : passing on knowledge

At the heart of professional progression in medicine is mentoring, a sacred process of passing on knowledge, skills and values from one generation to the next. In hematology, where the complexity of pathologies requires specialist expertise, mentoring is of paramount importance. It's not just a teaching method: it's an essential link in the chain of quality care, ensuring that every patient benefits from the accumulation of knowledge and past experience.

The Essence of Mentoring
Mentoring is not just about passing on information or demonstrating techniques. It is a deep relationship between mentor and mentee, based on trust, guidance and mutual support. The mentor doesn't just teach: he or she inspires, motivates and guides, helping the mentee to navigate the challenges of the profession and develop his or her own style and voice.

The benefits of mentoring
The benefits of mentoring are numerous and extend far beyond the acquisition of technical knowledge. The mentee benefits from an informed career perspective, help in avoiding common pitfalls and an extensive professional network. The mentor, meanwhile, benefits from an opportunity for reflection, a sense of achievement and a chance to leave a lasting legacy in the field.

Ongoing training
In addition to mentoring, continuing education plays a crucial role in hematology. With the rapid evolution of

knowledge, techniques and technologies, the need to keep up to date is imperative. This can take the form of online training, seminars, conferences or practical workshops.

Passing on knowledge beyond the hospital walls
The transmission of knowledge is not limited to the relationship between mentor and mentee. It extends to the community, patients and their families. Hematology nurses can play a pedagogical role, educating the public about the importance of donating blood, the signs and symptoms of haematological diseases, or the latest advances in treatment.

The Future of Mentoring and Training
With the advent of digital technologies, mentoring and training continue to evolve. Online platforms, virtual simulations and professional social networks offer new opportunities for learning and connecting. However, the intrinsic value of the human relationship in mentoring remains unrivalled.

Mentoring and training are two essential pillars in the field of hematology. They ensure not only that skills and knowledge are passed on with integrity, but also that the flame of passion, curiosity and dedication continues to burn in the hearts of each new generation of nurses.

Chapter 15:
SAMPLING TECHNIQUES
AND HEMATOLOGY ANALYSES

Blood samples:
techniques and best practice

Blood sampling is one of the most common procedures in the medical field. For hematology nurses, mastering this technique is essential. But beyond simply extracting blood, it's a process that requires deep understanding, impeccable precision and genuine empathy for the patient.

Background to blood sampling in hematology
In hematology, blood is much more than just a fluid that circulates through our bodies. It serves as a window on an individual's overall health, revealing clues about diseases such as leukaemia, anaemia, coagulation disorders and many others. Consequently, a blood sample taken correctly is the key to making an accurate diagnosis and devising an effective treatment plan.

Sampling techniques
- **Venipuncture**: This is the most common method. It involves using a needle to pierce a vein, usually in the arm, and drawing a certain amount of blood.
- **Capillary puncture**: This is often used for rapid tests, such as blood glucose. It involves pricking the fingertip or heel in infants.

Good Practices
- **Preparation of the patient** : Before sampling, the patient must be properly informed of the procedure. For some tests, specific instructions such as fasting may be necessary.

- **Hygiene**: Thorough disinfection of the puncture site is crucial to avoid infection.
- **Site selection**: It is important to choose an appropriate vein, usually the median vein of the elbow. If difficulties arise, other sites may be considered.
- **Puncture technique**: The puncture must be quick and precise to minimise discomfort.
- **Labelling and handling**: Each sample must be correctly labelled and handled with care to ensure reliable results.

Communication with the Patient
Although blood sampling is a routine procedure, it can be a source of anxiety for many patients. The human approach is therefore essential. Nurses need to reassure patients, explain each step and be attentive to their comfort throughout the procedure.

Blood sampling, which may seem simple, is a skill that combines technique and communication. In hematology, accuracy is paramount. Through continuous training, regular practice and genuine empathy for patients, nurses ensure that every sample taken makes a valuable contribution to the diagnosis and treatment of hematology diseases.

Interpreting blood tests in hematology

Interpreting blood tests is a crucial skill for hematology nurses. More than just numbers, blood tests provide a detailed picture of a patient's hematology health and help guide the diagnosis, treatment and monitoring of blood disorders.

The scope of blood tests

A blood test is a window on haematopoiesis - the process by which the body produces its blood cells. These tests reveal information about the three main components of blood: red blood cells, white blood cells and platelets.

The Main Blood Balance Indicators and Their Significance

- Blood count :
    - **Haemoglobin (Hb)**: Measures the blood's ability to carry oxygen. A low value may indicate anaemia.
    - **Haematocrit (Hct)** : The percentage of blood volume made up of red blood cells. It is useful for assessing blood density.
    - **Red blood cells (RBC):** Their number and shape can indicate a number of conditions, including thalassaemia or sickle cell anaemia.
    - **White blood cells (WBC)**: An increase may indicate an infection, while a decrease could indicate a bone marrow problem.
    - **Platelets** : Essential for coagulation. Low numbers can lead to bleeding, while high numbers can increase the risk of thrombosis.
- **Leukocyte count**: This details the different types of white blood cells, such as neutrophils, lymphocytes, monocytes, eosinophils and basophils. Their respective proportions can help diagnose various diseases, such as leukaemia.
- **Erythrocyte indices**: These, such as VGM (mean corpuscular volume) or CCMH (mean corpuscular haemoglobin concentration), give an indication of the size and haemoglobin content of the red blood cells, helping to classify anaemia.

Beyond the Figures: Clinical Interpretation

The real skill lies in the ability to interpret these figures in the overall clinical context of the patient. For example, an elevated WBC could indicate an infection, but in hematology it could also be a sign of leukaemia.

The limits of blood tests
Although blood tests provide a wealth of information, they are only one piece of the puzzle. They must be interpreted in conjunction with other tests, such as bone marrow biopsies, and the patient's clinical symptoms.

Interpreting a hematology blood test is both an art and a science. It's not just about understanding the numbers, but placing them in the wider context of the patient's condition, medical history and presenting symptoms. For hematology nurses, mastering this skill is essential to providing optimal care and collaborating effectively with the rest of the medical team.

Other specific samples: lumbar punctures, myelograms, etc.

Sampling in hematology is not limited to blood samples. Other sampling techniques are essential for diagnosing, monitoring and treating blood and bone marrow diseases. These procedures require not only careful technique, but also thorough preparation and communication with the patient.

Lumbar punctures
Lumbar puncture, or spinal tap, involves removing cerebrospinal fluid (CSF) from the subarachnoid space of the spinal column.
- **Indications**: These include the diagnosis and monitoring of certain leukaemias and lymphomas which can invade the central nervous system.

- **Procedure**: The patient is generally in the foetal lateral position, and after a local anaesthetic, a needle is inserted between the lumbar vertebrae.
- **Post-procedure care**: Monitoring for any signs of headache, infection or other complications is crucial.

Myelogram
This is a study of the fluid and cells in the bone marrow.
- **Indications**: Diagnosis of diseases such as leukaemia, lymphoma, bone marrow aplasia and other marrow diseases.
- **Procedure**: After a local anaesthetic, a needle is inserted into the bone (usually the pelvis) to take a sample of bone marrow.
- **Post-procedure care**: The puncture site may be painful. Watch for signs of infection or bleeding.

Bone marrow aspiration
Similar to a myelogram, but the sample is aspirated to obtain a bone marrow sample.
- **Indications**: Diagnosis and monitoring of diseases affecting blood cell production.
- **Procedure**: Often performed at the same time as a myelogram.
- **Post-procedure care**: Concerns are similar to those for myelogram.

Communication and Patient Preparation
These procedures can be a source of anxiety for patients. It is essential to inform the patient about what to expect, how long it will take, what it may feel like and the reason for the procedure. Good communication not only helps to reduce anxiety, but also to obtain the patient's cooperation, which is essential for safety and effectiveness.

Performing and understanding these specific samples is essential for hematology nurses. They play a decisive role in the diagnosis and management of hematology diseases, and require impeccable technique, meticulous preparation and post-procedure attention to ensure patient safety and comfort.

Chapter 16:
PALLIATIVE CARE IN HEMATOLOGY

Introduction to palliative care specific to hematology

Palliative care, although traditionally associated with the end of life, is in fact a holistic approach aimed at improving the quality of life of patients and their families in the face of the consequences of a life-threatening illness. In hematology, this approach is particularly important given the complexity and severity of many blood disorders.

Hematology covers a wide range of diseases, from anaemia to acute leukaemia. Although many hematology disorders are now treatable or even curable, some patients may not respond to standard treatments or may be diagnosed at an advanced stage. For these individuals, the focus is on quality of life rather than cure.

Palliative care in hematology is different in several ways. Firstly, the symptoms associated with blood diseases, such as fatigue, bone pain or bleeding, require special expertise. Complications, such as infections or haemorrhages, can develop rapidly and require immediate intervention.

Managing pain, which is often present in advanced hematology diseases, is essential. It may be due to the disease itself, as in the case of bone pain associated with leukaemia, or to treatment, such as post-chemotherapy pain.

Communication is also central. Talking openly with patients and their families about expectations, hopes and fears is vital. Hematology, with its intensive treatments and potential side-effects, raises many questions about quality of life, the length of treatment, and when to transition to purely palliative care.

Emotional and psychological care are an integral part of this approach. Hematology diseases can have a profound impact on self-image, role within the family and future aspirations. Supporting the patient through these challenges is as crucial as managing the physical symptoms.

Finally, palliative care in hematology must also take into account the specific needs of families. Hematology disease affects not only the patient, but also those around them. Family support, education and communication are essential to help everyone navigate through this difficult period.

Palliative care in hematology is a fusion of medical science, compassion and communication. It places the patient and family at the heart of decision-making, seeking to offer the best possible balance between fighting the disease and preserving quality of life.

Managing symptoms and pain

Managing symptoms and pain is a key part of hematology care, given the many challenges associated with blood disorders. Whether in response to the disease itself or the side effects of treatment, an individualised, multi-dimensional approach is essential.

Understanding symptoms :
Hematology encompasses a variety of diseases that can present with distinct symptoms. Anemias may cause fatigue and shortness of breath; bleeding or bruising may

occur with bleeding disorders; and bone pain, fever and night sweats may accompany blood cancers.

Pain assessment :
The first step to managing pain effectively is to assess it. Standardised assessment tools can help quantify pain, but it is equally crucial to understand its nature, location, what exacerbates or relieves it, and its impact on the patient's daily life.

Pharmacological strategies :
Most hematology patients will benefit from medication to manage their pain. Analgesics range from non-opioid drugs such as paracetamol or anti-inflammatories, to more potent opioids such as morphine. In the context of hematology conditions, it is essential to monitor drug interactions and effects on bone marrow.

Non-pharmacological approaches:
Non-drug methods such as physiotherapy, relaxation, acupuncture or cold/heat therapy can be very beneficial. These techniques can be used alone or in conjunction with medication to provide optimum relief.

Managing side effects:
Hematology treatments can cause a range of side effects, from nausea and hair loss to more serious complications such as heart failure or infection. Proactive management of these symptoms is vital to ensure the patient's well-being and ability to continue treatment.

Ongoing communication:
Effective symptom management depends on open and regular communication between the patient, their family and the healthcare team. Needs and symptoms can change, requiring ongoing adjustments to the management strategy.

Patient and family education:
It is essential that patients and their families understand the nature of the disease, what to expect in terms of symptoms and how to manage them. A well-informed patient is better able to participate actively in his or her own care.

Conclusion:
Managing symptoms and pain in hematology requires a combination of medical skills, compassion and communication. By putting the patient at the heart of this approach, carers can offer not only symptom relief but also a significant improvement in quality of life.

Psychological and spiritual support

In hematology, diagnosis, treatment, side-effects and associated uncertainties can have a considerable impact on patients' mental, emotional and spiritual well-being. Psychological and spiritual support is therefore of crucial importance.

The psychological dimension :
- **Impact of the diagnosis:** For many people, receiving a diagnosis in hematology can be overwhelming. Patients may feel overwhelmed, frightened or helpless in the face of the disease.
- **Psychological follow-up:** Healthcare professionals must be trained to recognise the signs of psychological distress. Specialist psychologists or psycho-oncologists may be required to help patients manage anxiety, depression or post-traumatic stress.
- **Support groups:** Support groups provide a space where patients and their families can share their experiences, learn from others and feel less isolated.

The spiritual dimension :
- **The need for meaning:** Faced with a serious illness, many patients wonder about the meaning of their lives, their raison d'être or the nature of their suffering.
- **Spiritual support:** Hospital chaplains or other spiritual advisors can provide support, whatever the patient's faith or belief. They offer a listening ear,

support with religious rites or simply a reassuring presence.

- **Rituals and traditions:** For some people, practising rituals or following traditions can offer comfort, structure and perspective in the face of illness.

Communication and education :

- **Open dialogue:** Carers should encourage patients to express their concerns and feelings, whether psychological or spiritual.
- **Tools and resources:** Providing patients with resources such as books, workshops or meditation sessions can help them navigate their emotions and questions.

The holistic approach to hematology is not limited to physical treatment. The psychological and spiritual dimensions are intrinsic to the healing process. By recognising and responding to these needs, carers can offer comprehensive care that respects every dimension of the human being. True healing goes beyond cells and tissues; it encompasses the mind, the soul and the heart.

Chapter 17:
COMPLEMENTARY THERAPIES AND ALTERNATIVES

Overview of approaches unconventional methods in hematology

Hematology, like many other medical specialities, has seen a growing interest in complementary and alternative therapies. These approaches, although unconventional, can often offer patients additional ways of managing their symptoms, stress and general well-being. Here is an overview of the unconventional approaches commonly explored in hematology.

Traditional medicines :
- **Acupuncture:** Originating in traditional Chinese medicine, acupuncture is sometimes used to manage pain, fatigue or nausea associated with certain hematology treatments.
- **Herbal supplements:** Although some herbs are beneficial, it is essential that patients inform their haematologist of any herbal supplements they are taking, as there may be interactions with their medication.

Mind-body methods :
- **Meditation and mindfulness:** These techniques can help to reduce stress, improve emotional well-being and increase pain tolerance.
- **Yoga and Tai Chi:** These forms of exercise can help improve flexibility, reduce fatigue and promote a general sense of well-being.

Nutrition and dietetics :
- **Special diets:** Some patients may explore specific diets in the hope of improving their health. It is always advisable to consult a nutritionist before making any significant changes to your diet.
- **Supplements and vitamins:** Although some can be beneficial, it is crucial to discuss them with a haematologist to avoid possible drug interactions.

Energy therapies :
- **Reiki: This is a** form of energy therapy in which the practitioner channels energy to help promote healing and well-being.
- **Biofeedback:** This technique enables patients to control certain physiological functions to improve their condition.

Unconventional approaches can offer many benefits for hematology patients. However, the key lies in balancing these therapies with conventional treatments. Open communication between the patient and his or her healthcare team is essential to ensure the safety and efficacy of the overall treatment plan.

Integration of alternative medicines: acupuncture, aromatherapy, etc.

In the age of modern medicine, more and more patients and healthcare professionals are turning to alternative therapies to complement or enhance traditional care. In hematology, the integration of these therapies can offer an additional dimension of care, focused on the patient's overall well-being.

Acupuncture :
Origins and principles: Originating in traditional Chinese medicine, acupuncture is based on the stimulation of

specific points on the body, generally using needles, to rebalance the flow of energy, or "Qi".

Applications in hematology: Hematology patients can benefit from acupuncture to manage pain, fatigue and post-chemotherapy nausea and vomiting. The effectiveness of this practice has been demonstrated in certain cases, although the exact mechanisms remain debated.

Aromatherapy :

Origins and principle: Aromatherapy uses essential oils extracted from plants to promote physical and mental health.

Applications in hematology: Used primarily for well-being, aromatherapy can help reduce anxiety, improve sleep and relieve certain ailments such as headaches. For hematology patients, it can be a non-invasive approach to complement conventional treatment.

Therapeutic massage :

Origins and principle: Massage is one of the oldest forms of therapy, used to release muscular tension, improve blood circulation and promote relaxation.

Applications in hematology: Gentle massage can help patients manage the pain and stress associated with their illness and treatment. However, it is crucial to choose a therapist trained in the specificities of hematology pathologies.

Meditation and mindfulness :

Origins and principle: These ancient practices aim to bring about a state of mental calm by concentrating on the present moment.

Applications in hematology: It can be particularly beneficial for patients suffering from anxiety or depression. Mindfulness can help to manage pain and live better with illness.

Integrating alternative medicine into hematology requires a balanced approach and open communication between the patient and the medical team. These therapies are not intended to replace conventional treatment, but rather to enrich it, by focusing on the patient's overall well-being, both physical and mental.

The nurse's role in guidance patients to these therapies

The nurse is often the first point of contact between the patient and the medical team, and this bond of trust established over the course of consultations and treatment makes his or her role essential in guiding patients towards complementary therapies.

1. Informed educator :
Nurses need to be informed about the different complementary therapies available and their potential benefits for the patient. This knowledge makes it possible to provide objective information, debunk myths and guide patients correctly according to their needs and preferences.

2. Active listening :
By actively listening to patients' concerns and wishes, nurses can identify those who might benefit from complementary therapies. They can also detect patients who are already turning to these approaches, sometimes without informing their medical team.

3. Connection point :
The nurse acts as a liaison between the patient and the medical team, ensuring that all parties are informed of decisions concerning complementary therapies. This guarantees comprehensive care, with no overlap or potential contraindications.

4. Emotional support :
The discovery and integration of new therapies into a care programme can be a source of anxiety and confusion for some patients. The nurse, by being close by and available,

can reassure, support and help patients understand the importance of each approach in their overall treatment.

5. Patient advocacy :

If the nurse is convinced of the benefits of a complementary therapy for a particular patient, he or she can discuss it with the medical team to see how it can be incorporated into the care plan.

6. Continuing education :

The world of complementary therapies is constantly evolving. To remain a reliable guide, nurses need to keep abreast of the latest research and trends, particularly through training courses and seminars.

7. Raising awareness :

Nurses can play a role in raising awareness among their colleagues and management, advocating wider integration of complementary therapies in the establishment or dedicated training courses.

The hematology nurse is much more than a provider of technical care: he or she is a guide, an adviser and a support. Their role in guiding patients towards complementary therapies is crucial to ensuring holistic care, centred on the patient's overall well-being, while ensuring consistency and safety of care.

Chapter 18:
SAFETY AND PREVENTION INFECTIONS

Prevention of nosocomial infections in hematology

Hematology departments cater for patients whose immune systems are often compromised, either by the disease itself or by the treatments administered, such as chemotherapy. These patients are therefore particularly vulnerable to nosocomial infections, making preventive measures crucial in these departments.

1. Understanding risk :
Before embarking on prevention, it is crucial to understand that hematology patients, as a result of their illness or treatment, have reduced immune defences, making them more susceptible to infection.

2. Hand hygiene :
This is the most basic and effective measure. Caregivers must wash their hands regularly, especially before and after contact with each patient. Hydro-alcoholic solution is a quick and effective way of doing this, but it must be used correctly.

3. Wearing personal protective equipment (PPE) :
Gloves, masks, gowns and other equipment must be used during procedures likely to expose carers and patients to infectious agents. This equipment must be changed between patients.

4. Patient isolation :
Some patients, particularly those with active infections, should be placed in isolation to prevent spread. Isolation can be reinforced for particularly vulnerable patients.

5. Staff training :

Staff must be regularly trained and informed about best practice in preventing nosocomial infections, including strict compliance with protocols.

6. Cleaning and disinfection :

Areas, particularly patient rooms, must be regularly cleaned and disinfected. Particular attention should be paid to frequently touched surfaces.

7. Monitoring :

It is essential to have a system for monitoring hospital-acquired infections, so that any outbreaks can be quickly identified and corrective action taken.

8. Controlled visits :

Limiting the number of visitors and ensuring they follow the same hygiene protocols as staff can help reduce the spread of infection.

9. Vaccinations :

Care staff should be up to date with their vaccinations to avoid transmitting diseases to patients. Similarly, if the patient's condition allows, it may be a good idea to vaccinate them against certain common infections.

10. Prevention of medical devices associated with infection :

Catheters, ventilators and other devices can be sources of infection if they are not properly managed. It is crucial to follow protocols for their insertion, maintenance and removal.

11. Nutrition :

A well-nourished patient is often better equipped to fight infection. Ensuring adequate nutrition can help strengthen a patient's immune system.

12. Raising awareness among patients and their families :
Patients and their families must be informed of the risks of infection and the measures they can take to protect themselves.

Preventing nosocomial infections in hematology requires a combination of education, strict protocols and constant monitoring. Collaboration between all healthcare staff is crucial to ensuring patient safety, and every measure, however basic, plays an essential role in preventing infections.

Universal precautions and specific

The safety of patients and healthcare professionals is a key concern in the medical sector. To avoid the transmission of infections, it is essential to adopt standardised preventive measures adapted to each situation. This is where universal and specific precautions come into their own.

1. Universal precautions :
These precautions apply to all patients, whatever their illness or diagnosis, because a patient's infectious status is not always known.
a. Hand hygiene :
This is the first line of defence against the spread of infections. Regular use of hydro-alcoholic solutions or hand washing with soap and water is essential.
b. Personal protective equipment (PPE):
The use of gloves, masks, goggles and coats should be routine where there is a risk of exposure to blood or other body fluids.
c. Safe handling of sharps:
Needles, scalpels and other sharp objects must be handled with care and disposed of in specific containers to avoid accidental punctures or cuts.

d. Medical waste management :
Waste must be sorted, packaged and disposed of in accordance with current standards to reduce the risk of contamination.

2. Specific precautions :
These precautions are implemented according to the mode of transmission of the infectious agent.
a. Droplet precautions :
These are necessary for diseases transmitted by respiratory droplets, such as influenza. The use of surgical masks and the establishment of a safe distance between the infected patient and others are recommended.
b. Contact precautions :
For diseases transmitted by direct or indirect contact, such as Staphylococcus aureus. Wearing gloves and gowns is recommended, as well as isolating the patient if necessary.
c. Airborne precautions :
These concern diseases such as tuberculosis, which are transmitted by very fine particles remaining suspended in the air. A negative pressure chamber and the use of FFP2 or N95 masks are essential.
d. Specific precautions for enteric diseases:
For diseases such as Clostridium difficile, enhanced hygiene measures and the use of chlorine solutions for cleaning are required.

Knowledge and rigorous application of universal and specific precautions are essential to protect both patients and healthcare staff. These measures, combined with ongoing training, can significantly reduce the risk of nosocomial infections and ensure safe, high-quality care for all patients.

The importance of vaccination in hematology patients

Hematology is a medical speciality that deals with diseases of the blood and the organs that produce it. Patients suffering from these diseases, whether leukaemia, lymphoma or other conditions, may have an increased susceptibility to infections as a result of their disease itself or the treatments they receive. In this context, vaccination is of particular importance in protecting these vulnerable patients.

1. A weakened immune system: a breeding ground for infection
In hematology patients, the immune system is often compromised, either by the disease itself or by treatments such as chemotherapy, radiotherapy or immunosuppressants. This vulnerability makes them more susceptible to infections, even those that would be benign to the general public.

2. Prevention as the first line of defence
Vaccination boosts the immune system against certain infections, offering essential protection. It reduces the risk of severe infections, hospitalisation and complications from vaccine-preventable diseases.

3. Specific vaccines for specific needs
Most vaccines can be administered to hematology patients, but care must be taken:
- **Live attenuated vaccines:** These vaccines are generally contraindicated in immunocompromised patients, as they may cause the disease they are intended to prevent.
- **Inactivated vaccines:** These are generally safe and are often strongly recommended for hematology

patients. They can protect against diseases such as influenza, pneumonia and hepatitis B.

4. Synchronisation is key
The optimal time to vaccinate a hematology patient often depends on the nature of the disease and its treatment. For example, it may be preferable to vaccinate before starting chemotherapy or between two cycles of treatment.

5. Those around you must also be protected
Relatives and carers of hematology patients should also be up to date with their vaccinations. This creates a "wall of protection" around the patient, reducing the chances of exposure to infection.

For hematology patients, vaccination is a valuable tool for minimising the risks associated with infections. With careful planning and close collaboration between the patient, the haematologist and the healthcare team, vaccination can offer robust protection, contributing to the safety and well-being of the patient's medical journey.

Chapter 19:
EMERGENCY MANAGEMENT IN HEMATOLOGY

Identify and act dealing with a bleeding emergency

A bleeding emergency is a life-threatening situation that requires rapid recognition and immediate intervention. In the context of hematology, patients may be at increased risk of bleeding due to underlying diseases or treatments that affect blood clotting. Here's an overview of how to identify and manage such an emergency.

1. Recognising the signs of haemorrhage
   * **External signs:** visible bleeding, often profuse, whether from a wound, natural orifices (nose, mouth, ears, rectum) or other sites.
   * **Internal signs:** pain or feeling of pressure, swelling, bruising, haematomas. In the case of gastrointestinal haemorrhage, Feces may be black and tarry or contain bright red blood.
   * **Systemic signs:** pallor, sweating, shortness of breath, tachycardia, hypotension, altered consciousness or dizziness.
2. Initial intervention
   * **Ensure safety:** Make sure the environment is safe for the patient and the care team.
   * **Positioning:** Lay the patient down, elevating the legs if possible, to encourage venous return.
   * **Controlling bleeding:** Apply direct pressure to the source of bleeding using a clean dressing or cloth. If necessary, use bandages or tourniquets for limb haemorrhages, but with caution and knowledge of their use.

3. Alert professionals
- **Call for help:** Immediately call an emergency team or specialist doctor.
- **Assessment: Once** the team is present, a rapid assessment of the cause of the haemorrhage, the volume of blood lost and the patient's haemodynamic stability is required.

4. Treatment and care
- **Volume resuscitation:** Administer fluids, generally saline or colloid solutions, to maintain adequate blood pressure and cardiac output.
- **Haemostatic drugs:** Depending on the cause, agents such as desmopressin, coagulation factors or platelets may be administered.
- **Transfusions :** Patients may require transfusion of red blood cells, platelets or other blood components.

5. Identify the cause and treat
- **Examination:** Imaging tests, such as ultrasound or CT scan, can help locate the source of the haemorrhage.
- **Interventions :** Surgical or endoscopic interventions may be necessary to stop active bleeding.

When faced with a haemorrhagic emergency, rapid and precise intervention is essential to save lives. Regular training, in-depth knowledge of hematology patients and close collaboration between the various healthcare professionals are crucial to ensuring the best possible care in these critical situations.

Chemotherapy emergencies

Chemotherapy, although essential in the treatment of many oncological and haematological conditions, is not without risks. It can give rise to a host of complications that can rapidly become medical emergencies. Understanding these emergencies and knowing how to respond to them is essential for all healthcare professionals working in hematology.

1. Allergic and anaphylactic reactions
   - **Presentation:** Redness, hives, facial swelling, difficulty breathing, hypotension.
   - **Intervention:** Immediate cessation of chemotherapy, administration of antihistamines, corticosteroids, or even adrenaline in the event of a severe reaction.
2. Capillary Leak Syndrome (CLS)
   - **Presentation:** Sudden oedema, weight gain, hypotension.
   - **Intervention:** Administration of corticosteroids and diuretics, adjustment of fluids and close monitoring.
3. Tumour lysis syndrome
   - **Presentation:** Hyperkalaemia, hyperuricaemia, hyperphosphataemia, acute renal failure.
   - **Intervention:** Hydration, alkalinisation of urine, administration of allopurinol or rasburicase.
4. Cardiac toxicity
   - **Presentation:** Dyspnoea, oedema, arrhythmias, chest pain.
   - **Intervention:** Electrocardiogram, echocardiography, discontinuation of the chemotherapy agent concerned, administration of cardio-protective agents.
5. Chemotherapy-induced pneumonitis
   - **Presentation:** Cough, dyspnoea, fever, hypoxia.
   - **Intervention:** Chest X-ray, discontinuation of chemotherapy agent, corticosteroids.
6. Peripheral neuropathy
   - **Presentation:** Numbness, tingling, pain, muscle weakness.
   - **Intervention:** Reduction of the dose or stopping the agent responsible, medication for neuropathic pain.

7. Hematology toxicity
- **Presentation:** Febrile neutropenia, anaemia, thrombocytopenia.
- **Intervention:** blood cultures, broad-spectrum antibiotics, transfusions, growth factors.

8. Dovetail syndrome
- **Description:** Blurred vision, high blood pressure, neurological disorders.
- **Intervention:** Cerebral imaging, reduction in intracranial pressure, corticosteroids.

Chemotherapy, although powerful and beneficial, presents undeniable challenges in terms of side effects and complications. The hematology nurse must be prepared to identify these emergencies quickly so that he or she can intervene appropriately, in close collaboration with the medical team, to ensure the patient's safety and well-being. Ongoing training and experience are essential to navigate these complex situations competently.

Rapid response protocols in hematology

Hematology is a rich and complex medical field where emergencies can arise suddenly. To ensure optimal patient care, it is vital that the medical team can rely on rapid intervention protocols. These protocols aim to standardise the response to critical situations, enabling effective, coordinated action.

1. Tumour lysis syndrome
- **Presentation:** Hyperkalaemia, hyperuricaemia, hyperphosphataemia, acute renal failure.
- **Protocol:** Intensive IV hydration, urine alkalinisation with sodium bicarbonate, administration of allopurinol or rasburicase, close renal and electrolyte monitoring.

2. Febrile neutropenia
   - **Presentation:** Temperature > 38°C with low neutrophil count.
   - **Protocol:** Rapid collection of blood cultures, immediate administration of broad-spectrum antibiotics, monitoring for signs of septic shock.
3. Bleeding emergencies
   - **Presentation:** Sudden, sometimes massive bleeding.
   - **Protocol:** Compression of bleeding areas, rapid blood transfusion (depending on the situation), administration of clotting factors or platelets, investigation of the underlying cause.
4. Transfusion reactions
   - **Presentation:** Fever, chills, pain, dyspnoea shortly after a transfusion.
   - **Protocol:** Stop transfusion, maintain IV line with saline, take blood cultures, check blood compatibility, monitor for signs of renal failure.
5. Vaso-occlusive crisis (sickle cell anaemia)
   - **Presentation:** Intense pain, oedema, fever.
   - **Protocol:** hydration, analgesia (often opioid-based), oxygen therapy if necessary, exchange transfusion in severe cases.
6. Thrombosis or embolism
   - **Presentation:** Pain, oedema, redness (venous thrombosis), sudden shortness of breath, chest pain (pulmonary embolism).
   - **Protocol:** Immediate anticoagulation, diagnostic imaging, bleeding monitoring.
7. Leukostasis (acute leukaemia)
   - **Presentation:** Dyspnoea, confusion, blurred vision.
   - **Protocol:** Hydration, possibly leukapheresis (filtration of white blood cells), induction chemotherapy in certain cases.

Rapid and effective intervention is essential in hematology to prevent serious complications. Rapid intervention protocols play a key role in giving patients the best possible chance of recovery. Ongoing training and regular simulations can help the medical team to remain ready and reactive to these emergencies.

Chapter 20:
ENVIRONMENT
AND SPECIFIC EQUIPMENT

The sterile room
and the negative pressure chamber

In hematology, some patients require care in environments specially designed to protect their health. This is particularly the case for patients who are immunocompromised or at risk of infection. Two types of chamber are particularly used in this context: the sterile chamber and the negative pressure chamber. Although they may appear similar at first glance, they meet different needs and have their own specific characteristics.

1. The sterile room: a protective bubble
- **Purpose:** It is designed to protect the patient from external infections. It is an environment where air, objects and people are sterilised to minimise the risk of introducing infectious agents.
- Features :
    - **Filtered air:** HEPA filters are used to eliminate particles and micro-organisms.
    - **Controlled entry and exit:** People entering the room must follow a strict protocol, including wearing sterile clothing and often taking an antiseptic shower.
    - **Constant monitoring:** Regular checks are carried out to ensure that the environment is sterile.
- **Indications :** Mainly used for patients who have undergone bone marrow transplantation or intensive chemotherapy, and are therefore in deep bone marrow aplasia.

2. The negative pressure chamber: a barrier against contaminants
- **Objective: To** prevent the spread of infectious agents outside the room, thereby protecting the rest of the hospital.
- Features :
  - **Negative pressure:** The air inside the chamber is constantly drawn towards a filtration system, preventing particles from escaping.
  - **Entrance airlock:** This prevents uncontrolled air movement between the room and the rest of the establishment.
  - **HEPA filters:** These purify the air leaving the chamber, eliminating potential pathogens.
- **Indications:** It is often used for patients suffering from airborne diseases such as tuberculosis or certain forms of influenza.

Conclusion

Each of these chambers plays a crucial role in the management of hematology patients. While the sterile room acts as a protective cocoon for the patient, the negative pressure room ensures that pathogens do not spread beyond the walls of the room. Mastery of the specific features and protocols associated with each chamber is essential for nurses, guaranteeing patient safety and well-being.

Use and maintenance hematology equipment

Hematology, at the crossroads between clinical research and practical care, requires the use of specific equipment, the performance of which is crucial for accurate diagnoses and appropriate management. Hematology nurses are often on the front line in the use of this equipment, whether for sampling, transfusion or analysis. Maintenance and control of these devices are therefore essential.

1. Centrifuges
Application: These machines are used to separate the different components of blood, such as plasma, platelets and red blood cells.
Maintenance: They must be cleaned regularly to avoid contamination. Checking the balance and replacing worn parts are also crucial.

2. Hematology analysers
Application: These automated devices count and classify blood cells, providing vital information about a patient's state of health.
Maintenance: Regular calibration, quality control and cleaning of the probes are essential to ensure accurate results.

3. Infusion pumps and transfusion devices
Use: These devices are used to administer drugs, blood or other fluids directly into a patient's circulatory system.
Maintenance: Tubing should be changed regularly, and equipment should be disinfected after each use.

4. Stem cell collection machines
Use: Used in stem cell transplants, these machines separate and collect stem cells from peripheral blood.
Maintenance: Rigorous sterilisation is necessary to prevent infection, and regular maintenance ensures optimum performance.

5. Refrigerators and freezers for blood storage
Use: To store blood products safely before use.
Maintenance: They should be checked daily to ensure that the temperature ranges are respected. In addition, regular cleaning prevents the proliferation of bacteria.

The hematology nurse plays a fundamental role in the use and maintenance of equipment, ensuring not only that care runs smoothly but also that patients are safe. A thorough understanding of each piece of equipment, combined with rigorous maintenance procedures, enables high quality care to be provided while minimising risks. This balance can only be maintained through ongoing training, updating of skills and close collaboration with the technical teams.

Technology and digitisation in hematology : advances and implications for nurses

The era of digitalization has opened the door to a multitude of innovations in the medical field. Hematology, like other specialties, has benefited from these advances, turning the traditional role of the nurse on its head. Technology has made possible what was once unthinkable, changing both the way nurses interact with patients and the way they manage their day-to-day responsibilities.

1. Telemedicine :

Telemedicine enables nurses to monitor patients with hematology diseases remotely, especially when they are at home. Using dedicated applications, patients can report their symptoms, providing a means of real-time monitoring and early intervention in the event of complications.

2. Patient management applications and platforms :

These digital platforms centralise patient information, including their medical history, current medication and laboratory tests. The nurse can access this information instantly, improving the efficiency of care.

3. Portable patient monitoring devices :
From smartwatches to connected bracelets, these devices can monitor heart rate, blood pressure and other vital indicators, alerting the nurse and care team to any potentially worrying changes.

4. Robots in hematology :
Certain processes, such as the mixing and preparation of chemotherapy drugs, are now automated, reducing errors and ensuring greater patient safety.

5. Virtual reality (VR) :
It is used to train hematology nurses. Thanks to VR, they can train in procedures without endangering a real patient.

6. Artificial intelligence and data analysis :
AI algorithms can help detect anomalies in blood tests or anticipate risks to the patient, helping nurses to make informed decisions.

Implications for nurses :
While these innovations offer many advantages, they also raise challenges for the hematology nurse. Ongoing training is essential if these new technologies are to be mastered. What's more, although digitalisation facilitates many processes, it cannot replace the human touch, empathy and face-to-face communication that remain at the heart of the nursing profession.

The intersection of technology and digitalisation with hematology has undoubtedly reshaped the medical landscape, offering valuable tools to improve patient care. However, as these advances continue to evolve, it is imperative that nurses remain at the centre of care, using technology as a tool and not as a replacement for their expertise and compassion.

Chapter 21:
INTERNATIONAL PERSPECTIVES AND COMPARATIVE

Hematology care: variations from country to country

Medicine is a universal discipline, but its application and access can vary considerably from one country to another. Hematology care is no exception, and is influenced by factors such as health policy, economics, culture and even a country's history. Let's explore how these elements shape hematology care around the world.

1. Availability of medical resources :
   - In developed countries, hospitals and clinics are often equipped with the latest technology, enabling early detection and treatment of hematology diseases.
   - Conversely, in developing countries, there may be a lack of advanced diagnostic equipment, which can delay diagnosis and treatment.
2. Access to medicines :
   - Some countries, particularly those with robust healthcare systems, have wide and rapid access to the latest drugs.
   - Others, because of financial or bureaucratic constraints, may not have access to these drugs or may receive them with considerable delay.
3. Training and education :
   - Countries with strong medical education systems produce highly qualified hematology specialists.
   - In regions where training is less accessible, there may be a shortage of specialists, which can affect the quality of care.

4. Tradition and alternative medicine :
   - In many cultures, traditional or alternative approaches may be favoured before or in conjunction with modern medicine.
   - Understanding and respecting these choices is crucial to providing holistic care.
5. Health policy :
   - Government policies greatly influence how hematology care is delivered. For example, some countries may have universal screening programmes for certain hematology diseases.
   - Others, because of budget restrictions or other priorities, may not offer these services.
6. Economics and financing :
   - Hematology treatment, especially with advanced therapies, can be expensive. In countries with a universal healthcare system or solid insurance, patients generally have fewer financial worries.
   - Elsewhere, cost can be a major barrier to access to healthcare.

Hematology care is a mirror reflecting the complexities and inequalities of the global medical world. While some patients benefit from the latest advances in diagnosis and treatment, others struggle to access even the most basic care. Recognising this diversity is the first step in building a world where quality hematology care is a reality for everyone, regardless of geography or wealth.

International best practice in hematology

Hematology, like any other medical field, is constantly evolving through research, technological innovation and international collaboration. Best practices" are strategies or techniques based on scientific evidence, which have been shown to be the most effective in patient management.

These practices may vary from region to region, but certain standards are recognised and adopted worldwide. Let's explore these best practices in hematology together.

1. Evidence-based treatment protocols :
   - The importance of randomised clinical trials and meta-analysis in determining the effectiveness of treatments.
   - Constant updating of treatment guidelines in line with new discoveries.
2. Early diagnosis and screening :
   - Use of advanced techniques, such as next-generation sequencing, to detect specific mutations and personalise treatment.
   - Screening programmes for groups at risk of certain hematology diseases.
3. Multidisciplinary approach :
   - Close collaboration between haematologists, oncologists, radiologists, pathologists and other specialists to ensure comprehensive patient care.
   - Regular multidisciplinary consultation meetings to discuss complex cases.
4. Patient-centred care :
   - Ensuring transparent communication with patients and their families, educating them about the disease and treatment.
   - Take into account the patient's psychological, social and emotional needs.
5. Continuing education :
   - Encouraging ongoing training for healthcare professionals to keep abreast of the latest advances.
   - Participation in international conferences, seminars and training courses.
6. Research and participation in clinical trials :
   - Promoting the importance of clinical research to discover new treatments or improve existing approaches.

- Establish international collaborations for large-scale trials.
7. Safety and quality of care :
   - Use of standardised protocols to minimise errors.
   - Regular monitoring of side effects and implementation of strategies to manage them.
8. Access to healthcare :
   - Ensuring that all patients, regardless of their socio-economic situation, have access to high-quality care.
   - Working with NGOs and other organisations to facilitate access to medicines and treatments in less privileged regions.

Best practice in hematology is the result of years of research, collaboration and dedication by the world's medical community. Adopting these practices not only ensures better patient care, but also a constant advance in the understanding and treatment of haematological diseases. In a globalised world, collaboration and the exchange of expertise are essential to continue improving care for all patients, wherever they may be.

International exchanges and cooperation for hematology nurses

The world of hematology is a constantly evolving one, where every discovery and advance pushes back the boundaries of what we know and what we can achieve. For hematology nurses, being at the heart of these advances is not just a question of keeping up to date with techniques and protocols. It's also an opportunity to build bridges, share knowledge, and enrich our practice through interactions with professionals from around the world.

Globalisation and technological advances have brought healthcare professionals closer together than ever before.

The exchange of skills, methodologies and experiences among hematology nurses from one nation to another has become commonplace, but it's much more than that. It's a symbiosis that allows each participant to grow, learn and contribute to a common goal: the best possible care for patients.

Many programmes and institutions around the world offer exchange opportunities for nurses. These programmes not only allow nurses to observe how hematology care is delivered in other cultures and healthcare systems, but also to share their own knowledge and perspectives. The differences between healthcare systems, cultural approaches to illness and care, and innovative techniques used elsewhere can offer valuable insights that enrich and diversify the practice of every nurse.

But these exchanges are not one-sided. The hematology nurses who take part in such programmes also contribute by bringing their expertise and unique perspective to their hosts. They become ambassadors for their own institutions and countries, sharing best practices, successful protocols and lessons learned.

In addition to formal exchanges, international hematology conferences offer opportunities for networking and collaboration. These events bring together the brightest minds in the field, allowing for in-depth discussion, debate and collaboration on studies and research projects. For a hematology nurse, attending such conferences is an invaluable opportunity to broaden their professional horizons, meet peers from different parts of the world and immerse themselves in the latest advances in the field.

Beyond knowledge and skills, what these exchanges and cooperative ventures bring above all is mutual understanding. They are a reminder that, whatever the distance or cultural differences, the core of the nursing profession remains the same: compassion, dedication and commitment to the well-being of patients.

So, through these international collaborations, hematology nurses are doing more than just honing their skills. They forge links, establish collaborations and, together, push back the frontiers of what is possible in hematology, for the benefit of patients around the world.

Chapter 22:
PREVENTION AND PROMOTION HEALTH IN HEMATOLOGY

Awareness campaigns blood diseases

Raising awareness is a powerful tool for educating, informing and inspiring concrete action in favour of a cause. In the case of blood disorders, raising awareness can not only help to detect and treat these diseases earlier, but also demystify certain preconceived ideas and provide support for patients and their families.

1. Why is awareness-raising crucial?
There are many hematology conditions, some common and others rarer. However, despite their prevalence, general knowledge of these diseases can be limited. Raising awareness helps to :
   • Recognising early symptoms.
   • Encourage regular screening.
   • Demystifying blood diseases.
   • Raising awareness of blood and bone marrow donation.
   • Promoting research and funding.

2. Key players in awareness-raising
It's not surprising that healthcare professionals, patients, their families and associations are at the forefront of awareness-raising efforts. Together, they create targeted campaigns, organise events and mobilise the media to bring the message to a wider audience.

3. Types of awareness campaigns
   • **Specific awareness days or months**: such as World Thalassaemia Day or Leukaemia Awareness Month,

these dedicated periods are ideal times to step up communication and education efforts.
- **Blood and bone marrow donation campaigns**: Encouraging the public to donate is essential for many patients suffering from blood diseases.
- **Conferences and workshops**: aimed at healthcare professionals, patients and the general public, these educational events cover recent advances, current challenges and hopes for the future.
- **Action in schools and universities**: Educating young people about blood diseases can help promote healthy habits and encourage the next generation to get involved.

4. The role of social media

Platforms such as Facebook, Twitter and Instagram have become invaluable tools for raising awareness. Personal stories, up-to-date information and online challenges can quickly reach and engage a wide audience.

5. Measuring the impact

Measuring the effectiveness of campaigns is crucial to ensure that resources are used wisely and that the message reaches its target. Feedback, surveys, social media analysis and blood donation data can provide valuable information.

Raising awareness of blood disorders is an ongoing effort that requires the collaboration, passion and dedication of everyone involved. Every initiative, large or small, contributes to a better future for those affected by these conditions.

Promoting blood donations and bone marrow

Donating blood and bone marrow is essential for many patients suffering from hematology diseases. These donations give a second chance at life, support vital treatments and promote research. However, despite its importance, there is still an urgent need for donors. Promoting these donations is therefore crucial to closing the gap between supply and demand.

1. The importance of donations
   - **Saving lives**: A single blood donation can help up to three patients, and a bone marrow donation may be the only chance of survival for a patient suffering from leukaemia or other blood diseases.
   - **Supporting medical treatment**: Blood transfusions are commonly used in many medical procedures, from major surgery to cancer treatment.
   - **Research and development**: Blood donations also contribute to medical research, paving the way for new discoveries and treatments.
2. Demystifying the donation process
   - **Safety first and foremost**: Blood and bone marrow donation procedures are strictly regulated to guarantee the safety of both donor and recipient.
   - **The process**: Educating the public about what to expect, how long it will take and how they will be looked after can help to dispel fears or misunderstandings.
3. Awareness campaigns
   - **Special donation days**: Organise days dedicated to blood and bone marrow donation in hospitals, universities and other institutions.
   - **Testimonials**: The stories of people who have benefited from bone marrow transfusions or

transplants can have a powerful emotional impact and motivate potential donors.

- **Media partnerships**: Working with radio stations, television channels and newspapers to broadcast awareness-raising messages.

4. Mobilising young people

Young adults are often in excellent health, which makes them particularly suitable for donation. Raising their awareness from an early age can create a culture of giving that continues into adulthood.

- **Campaigns in schools and universities**: Workshops, conferences or donation days can be organised to encourage students to donate.
- **Youth ambassadors**: Nominate motivated students to promote giving among their peers.

5. Post-donation support

Recognising and thanking donors is essential to encourage repeat donations.

- **Certificates and recognition**: Offer certificates or badges to recognise the donor's contribution.
- **Follow-up and care**: Follow-up after donation to ensure that the donor feels well and is ready to donate again.

Promoting blood and bone marrow donation requires a concerted effort from society as a whole. It's a cause that has the power to connect individuals, bring communities together and save lives. And every donation counts. Every gesture makes a difference.

The role of the nurse in prevention programmes

Nurses play a central role in public health. As the linchpin of the healthcare system, they are involved not only in curative care, but also in prevention. Prevention programmes are designed to educate, raise awareness and help people adopt healthy behaviours in order to avoid the onset or progression of disease. Nurses play several key roles in this context:

1. Health educator :
Nurses inform patients about the risks associated with certain illnesses, the behaviour to adopt and the actions to avoid. They give practical advice, demonstrate techniques (for example, how to wash your hands properly) and provide educational resources.

2. Health promoter :
As well as simply providing information, nurses actively encourage people to look after their health, whether through vaccinations, regular screening or adopting a healthy lifestyle.

3. Evaluator :
Nurses carry out health checks, identify potential risks for each individual and refer patients to specialists if necessary. They may also carry out screening tests in certain cases.

4. Care coordinator :
As part of prevention programmes, nurses often work in collaboration with other health professionals. In this way, they ensure optimum coordination of care for the patient, facilitating access to the necessary resources and providing regular follow-up.

5. Consultant :
Faced with sometimes complex medical decisions, nurses offer support and sound advice to patients, helping them to make informed choices about their health.

6. Patient advocate :
Nurses defend patients' rights and ensure that they receive appropriate care without discrimination. They may also play an active role in raising public awareness of certain health issues.

7. Researcher :
In some cases, nurses may take part in studies and research aimed at improving prevention programmes, by analysing their effectiveness and suggesting improvements.

8. Trainer :
Nurses may be called upon to train other health professionals or members of the community in preventive practices.

Nurses play a key role in prevention programmes. Their proximity to patients, their medical expertise and their ability to work as part of a team give them a unique role in the promotion of global and sustainable health. They work every day to improve the quality of life for all, by preventing rather than curing.

Chapter 23:
CULTURAL ASPECTS AND DIVERSITY

Understanding and respecting
the cultural diversity of patients

In today's interconnected world, carers, and nurses in particular, are frequently in contact with patients from diverse cultural backgrounds. Understanding and respecting these cultural differences is not only an ethical necessity, it is also crucial to providing appropriate and effective care.

When we talk about cultural diversity, we are not just referring to ethnicity or nationality, but also to religion, sexual orientation, age, gender, disability and many other factors that shape a person's identity and life experiences. Each individual has their own history, beliefs, values and practices, which can influence their perception of illness, well-being and medical care.

Taking the time to understand a patient's cultural context can have a significant impact on the outcome of care. For example, some patients may have dietary restrictions linked to their religious beliefs, or different views on medical interventions based on their cultural experiences. If these nuances are not recognised and respected, it can lead to misunderstandings, dissatisfaction and, more seriously, medical errors.

Communication is at the heart of this understanding. This means listening actively, asking open questions and never assuming that you know a patient's needs or preferences simply by their appearance or name. Carers must also be aware of their own prejudices and strive to set them aside when interacting with patients.

Respect for cultural diversity goes beyond mere tolerance. It means recognising and valuing differences as assets. It may mean learning a few key words in another language, becoming familiar with the customs and traditions of a particular culture, or finding out about traditional remedies that patients might use alongside Western treatments.

It is also important to remember that, while the Western medical approach has its merits, it is not the only route to recovery. Integrating and valuing traditional or complementary practices, where appropriate, can not only improve the effectiveness of care, but also strengthen trust between patient and carer.

Ultimately, the key lies in creating an inclusive care space, where each patient is seen and treated as a unique individual, with their own history, beliefs and needs. In such an environment, patients are more likely to feel understood, respected and cared for holistically, leading to better outcomes for all.

Cultural impact on beliefs and health-related behaviour

Culture is a set of values, beliefs, customs and practices that influence the way people perceive and interact with the world around them. When it comes to health, culture plays a dominant role, shaping beliefs, behaviours and attitudes towards illness, treatment, cure and even prevention. These cultural influences can vary considerably from one community to another and even within particular communities.

- **Conceptions of illness**: In many cultures, illness is not seen simply as a biological or physiological dysfunction. It may be seen as the result of an

143

energetic imbalance, divine punishment, possession by spirits or misalignment with natural forces. For example, some cultures believe that evil spirits or the evil eye can cause illness.

- **Therapeutic approaches**: Treatments vary according to cultural beliefs. While Western medicine focuses on drugs and surgery, other cultures may favour herbal medicine, acupuncture, prayer, meditation or spiritual rituals.
- **Roles and responsibilities**: In some cultures, the family plays a central role in healthcare decision-making, while in others the individual may be the main decision-maker. Similarly, traditional gender roles can influence who makes decisions and how healthcare is perceived.
- **Health communication**: The way symptoms are described, the preference for direct or indirect disclosure of medical information, and even pain tolerance can be influenced by cultural factors.
- **Attitudes towards healthcare professionals**: In some cultures, doctors and other healthcare professionals are regarded with immense respect and may not be questioned, while in others patients may prefer alternative treatments or traditional healers.
- **Preventive behaviours**: Cultural perceptions of health and illness can influence participation in preventive behaviours, such as vaccination, regular check-ups or even diet and exercise.

It is essential that healthcare professionals recognise and respect these diverse cultural beliefs and behaviours in order to provide patient-centred care. An approach that does not take into account the patient's culture may not only be ineffective, but also potentially harmful. By understanding and integrating the patient's cultural perspective, carers can build a relationship of trust, improving the effectiveness of care and patient satisfaction.

Strategies for appropriate and inclusive care

The cultural, ethnic and social diversity of patients requires an approach to care that recognises and values these differences. Healthcare professionals must strive to provide care that is tailored to each individual, taking into account their cultural background and specific needs. Here are some strategies for achieving this:

- **Intercultural training**: Encourage ongoing training for healthcare professionals to enable them to understand the various beliefs, values and practices that can influence patients' medical decisions.
- **Active communication**: Learning intercultural communication skills, such as active listening, reformulation and seeking feedback, to ensure that information is properly understood.
- **Interpreting services**: In multilingual areas, access to qualified interpreters or translation tools to ensure clear communication between healthcare professionals and patients.
- **Networking with the community**: Working with community leaders or organisations to understand and respect the specific needs and beliefs of each group.
- **Inclusive resources**: Educational material adapted to different cultural and linguistic groups, with relevant illustrations and examples.
- **Individual assessment**: Avoid generalising or stereotyping. Ask open and respectful questions to understand each patient's individual needs and preferences.

- **Holistic approach**: Recognising that health encompasses physical, mental, emotional and spiritual well-being. Take all these aspects into account when providing care.
- **Patient and family involvement**: Actively involving patients and their families in the decision-making process, respecting their beliefs and choices.
- **Adaptability**: Being flexible in therapeutic approaches, considering alternative or complementary treatments where appropriate and safe for the patient.
- **Peer support**: Encouraging exchanges between patients from the same cultural background or with similar experiences to share advice and coping strategies.
- **Review and continuous improvement**: Regularly evaluate the effectiveness of interventions and feedback from patients to ensure that care is appropriate and inclusive.
- **Creating a welcoming environment**: Elements such as multilingual signage, culturally diverse decoration and even music can help create an environment in which patients feel valued and comfortable.

Adapted and inclusive care is based on respect, understanding and compassion. By implementing these strategies, healthcare professionals can provide high-quality care that meets the unique needs of each patient, while honouring and valuing their cultural identity.

Chapter 24:
THE FUTURE OF HEMATOLOGY AND THE CHALLENGES AHEAD

New technologies and innovations in hematology

Medicine is constantly evolving, and has always benefited from the advent of new technologies. Hematology, the study of blood disorders, is no exception to this trend. Recent years have seen some remarkable innovations that are transforming the way we diagnose, treat and manage blood disorders.

- **Next-generation genomic sequencing**: Genomic sequencing enables exhaustive detection of genetic mutations that could be the cause of various blood diseases. This information can be used to develop personalised treatments.
- **Targeted therapies**: Using molecular genetics, it is now possible to create drugs that specifically target diseased cells, thereby reducing the side effects associated with more global therapies.
- **Immunotherapy**: CAR-T therapies, for example, modify the patient's own immune cells so that they target and attack cancer cells.
- **Liquid biopsy**: This method detects cancer cells or tumour DNA fragments circulating in the blood, offering a less invasive alternative to traditional biopsy.
- **Microfluidics**: Devices that manipulate small volumes of fluid can rapidly analyse blood cells and detect diseases.
- **Gene-editing technologies, such as CRISPR-Cas9**: These tools make it possible to

modify or 'correct' certain genetic mutations and have therapeutic potential in diseases such as sickle cell anaemia.

- **Information systems and artificial intelligence**: With the development of Big Data, algorithms can now help with diagnosis, the analysis of blood samples and the prediction of therapeutic responses.
- **Wearable tech**: Wearable devices can continuously monitor certain parameters, such as blood coagulation, and transmit this data in real time to healthcare professionals.
- **Gene therapies:** Techniques aimed at introducing or modifying genetic information within a patient's cells to treat a disease.
- **Transcranial Magnetic Stimulation (TMS)**: Used in the treatment of depression, research is underway to explore its potential usefulness in hematology disorders linked to bone marrow.
- **Nanotechnology**: The use of nanoparticles to administer drugs directly to diseased cells or to improve imaging.

These innovations, while promising, require further study to ensure their long-term efficacy and safety. Nevertheless, they offer the hope of significant improvements in the diagnosis, treatment and management of blood diseases in the future. By integrating these technologies into clinical practice, haematologists can look forward to improved outcomes and a better quality of life for their patients.

The challenges of ageing of the population

The demographic transition towards a world where a significant proportion of the population is elderly is an increasingly marked phenomenon. This ageing of the population is the result of a combination of two factors: increased life expectancy thanks to medical progress and a fall in the birth rate in many parts of the world. Although this is often seen as a success story for our modern societies, the ageing of the population brings with it its own set of challenges and issues.

One of the key issues is **health**. Older people are more likely to suffer from a wide range of chronic conditions requiring prolonged medical care. The prevalence of degenerative diseases such as Alzheimer's, Parkinson's and various forms of arthritis increases with age. As a result, healthcare systems need to adapt to meet the growing demand for specialist and home care.

The ageing of the population also has **economic repercussions**. Once retired, older people depend mainly on their pensions or savings to live on. With a growing proportion of the population no longer working, current pension systems, often based on pay-as-you-go, could come under pressure. The question of the sustainability of pensions is therefore becoming crucial.

From a **social perspective**, demographic ageing is also changing the dynamics of families and communities. Intergenerational solidarity is put to the test as younger generations often have to reconcile their own professional and family obligations with caring for their elders.

Urban planning and **regional development** are also being affected. Towns and cities need to rethink their infrastructure to make it more accessible to the elderly: adapted public transport, safe urban development, adapted and accessible housing, and public spaces designed for everyone.

Finally, there is a cultural issue. In many cultures, older people are seen as the repositories of wisdom and history.

However, in a constantly changing world, marked by digital technology and technological revolutions, the **place and role of** senior citizens in society may be called into question.

Faced with these challenges, we need to rethink our social, economic and health models. Adapting to this new demographic reality requires a holistic approach, involving all players in society, from the public to the private sector, and including civil society. The challenge is immense, but it also offers the opportunity to build a more inclusive world, where each generation finds its place and makes its contribution.

Looking ahead : the hematology of tomorrow

Hematology, the medical branch dedicated to the study of blood, its diseases and their treatment, has made enormous strides in recent decades. Today, thanks to the convergence of technology, research and clinical practice, we are at the dawn of a new era for this speciality. Looking to the future of hematology, we see a world where medicine is more precise, personalised, preventive and participatory.

1. Personalised medicine: The genomic revolution has already begun to transform the treatment of hematology diseases. Patients are no longer categorised simply by the symptoms of their disease, but by their unique genetic profile. This enables a tailor-made approach, where treatments are specifically designed according to the patient's genetics, increasing efficacy and reducing side effects.

2. Advanced therapies: Cellular therapies, such as CAR-T therapy, in which the patient's own cells are modified to attack cancer cells, are gaining ground. Although expensive, these treatments have shown remarkable success rates for certain blood cancers previously considered incurable.

3. Improved diagnosis: Technology is making it possible to obtain increasingly precise images of the human body. This means that diagnoses can be made faster and more accurately. What's more, artificial intelligence and machine learning could help clinicians detect diseases at a much earlier stage.

4. Proactive prevention: With a better understanding of genetic and environmental risk factors, we may be able to identify individuals at risk of developing certain hematology diseases and intervene well before the first symptoms appear.

5. Patient involvement : Technological advances, such as health applications and connected objects, could enable patients to monitor their own state of health, understand their illness and play a more active role in their treatment.

6. Global collaboration: Diseases know no borders, and neither does science. Tomorrow's hematology will be characterised by unprecedented collaboration between researchers, clinicians and patients from all over the world. This collaboration could accelerate research, the discovery of treatments and the dissemination of best practice on a global scale.

7. Ethics and equity: With the advent of costly new therapies, the question of equitable access to treatment for all patients, regardless of their place of residence or socio-economic situation, will arise. Ethical reflection will be essential to ensure that progress benefits everyone.

Tomorrow's vision of hematology is of a medical speciality in the throes of change, driven by innovation and collaboration. It promises a future where blood diseases can be not only treated but also prevented, where every patient is a player in his or her own health, and where medicine is fairer and more equitable. The road to this vision will be fraught with challenges, but the possibilities are endless.

www.ingramcontent.com/pod-product-compliance
Lightning Source LLC
Chambersburg PA
CBHW072209290526
45794CB00004B/1701